The TEN KEYS
to Helping Your
Child *Grow Up*
with DIABETES

Tim Wysocki, PHD

Director, Book Publishing, John Fedor; *Associate Director, Consumer Books,* Sherrye Landrum, *Editor,* Abe Ogden; *Associate Director, Book Production,* Peggy M. Rote; *Composition and cover Design,* Circle Graphics; *Printer,* Worzalla Publishing Co.

Printed in the United States of America
1 3 5 7 9 10 8 6 4 2

The suggestions and information contained in this publication are generally consistent with the *Clinical Practice Recommendations* and other policies of the American Diabetes Association, but they do not represent the policy or position of the Association or any of its boards or committees. Reasonable steps have been taken to ensure the accuracy of the information presented. However, the American Diabetes Association cannot ensure the safety or efficacy of any product or service described in this publication. Individuals are advised to consult a physician or other appropriate health care professional before undertaking any diet or exercise program or taking any medication referred to in this publication. Professionals must use and apply their own professional judgment, experience, and training and should not rely solely on the information contained in this publication before prescribing any diet, exercise, or medication. The American Diabetes Association—its officers, directors, employees, volunteers, and members—assumes no responsibility or liability for personal or other injury, loss, or damage that may result from the suggestions or information in this publication.

∞ The paper in this publication meets the requirements of the ANSI Standard Z39.48-1992 (permanence of paper).

ADA titles may be purchased for business or promotional use or for special sales. To purchase this book in large quantities, or for custom editions of this book with your logo, contact Lee Romano Sequeira, Special Sales & Promotions, at the address below, or at LRomano@diabetes.org or 703-299-2046.

American Diabetes Association
1701 North Beauregard Street
Alexandria, Virginia 22311

Library of Congress Cataloging-in-Publication Data
Wysocki, Tim, 1949-
   Ten keys to helping your child grow up with diabetes / Tim Wysocki.—2nd ed.
     p. cm.
   Includes bibliographical references and index.
   ISBN 1-58040-186-4 (pbk. : alk. paper)
     1. Diabetes in children—Popular works. 2. Diabetes in children—Patients—Care. I. Title.
RJ420.D5W97 2004
362.1'9892462—dc22

                                               2003063658

CONTENTS

PREFACE

t's hard to believe that 7 years have already passed since the first edition of this book went to press. During that time, much about living and coping with childhood diabetes has changed, but much has also remained the same. In this second edition, I've tried to retain what I see as the strengths of this book: a focus on 10 key tasks faced by young people with diabetes and their parents; the presentation of a wide variety of practical solutions and approaches to those challenges; and a basis in effective coping techniques obtained through careful scientific research. At the same time, I've tried to revise the book to keep pace with modern advances in scientific knowledge about diabetes, its causes, and its treatment. Among the main changes that you may notice in the second edition are:

▲ Greater emphasis on type 2 diabetes, which has become an epidemic in children and adolescents since the first edition of this book was published.

▲ Increased attention to the special issues facing families of infants, toddlers, and preschoolers with diabetes.

▲ More discussion of diabetes management regimens such as the use of insulin pumps, carbohydrate counting, and other such medical advances.

▲ Greater recognition that the modern "family" varies greatly, and that diabetes educational materials must be relevant to families with diverse ethnic, economic, and structural characteristics.

▲ Addition of "For Fathers Only" sections to several chapters. Recent research has shown how important the contribution of fathers is to child development and the prevention of many adverse outcomes during adolescence.

During the past 23 years, I have devoted most of my professional life to working as a pediatric psychologist with families such as yours who are trying their best to raise a child or adolescent with diabetes in the safest, healthiest, and most satisfying way possible. In this time, I have recognized that parents and caregivers of children with diabetes need a practical guide that would help them do the best possible job in their most important role.

There are already wonderful books that can give you excellent and practical medical and nutritional information about childhood diabetes and its treatment (see the reading list in the "Resources" section), but none talk in length about the psychological, social, and emotional hurdles that often complicate the lives of youngsters with diabetes. These are commonly the most pressing concerns of parents, young people with diabetes, and health care providers, yet our typical medical and educational approaches often neglect to talk about the skills you need to deal with them effectively.

In the past two decades, more and more diabetes teams have come to include mental health professionals, such as psychologists, psychiatrists, social workers, and counselors. Although we are a still a long way from having proper access to such services for all families living with diabetes, the situation is slowly improving and I am hopeful that this will continue. During this time, research on the psychological, behavioral, and emotional aspects of diabetes has also expanded greatly. There are now several thousand published research studies on the psychological aspects of childhood diabetes alone. I have drawn extensively on this research in writing this book, and I list the references to many of the most important studies in the Resources section. I've done my best to represent the consensus of opinion among psychologists, psychiatrists, and other behavioral scientists who are experts on childhood diabetes. Although delving into research articles may be beyond your level of interest, I wanted to make it possible for all readers to appreciate the strong scientific bases for the main points made in the book.

Even when the services of psychologists, psychiatrists, counselors, or social workers are available, it may be hard to make use of them. These services may not be sought until a crisis arises, it may not be possible to find a mental health professional who knows about diabetes, insurance coverage may be limited, you may feel embarrassed about seeking help with mental health, and the current health care system generally doesn't pay for preventive mental health services. Also, doctors and nurses may not be totally aware of a family's need for help in these areas, and so it often falls to you to ask for a referral to a psychologist, psychiatrist, or mental health counselor.

In writing this book, I've tried to stress the need for a broader approach to helping more families with the psychological aspects of diabetes. You need to understand the psychological impact of the disease, learn practical solutions to some of the common hurdles that you and your child may encounter, and have a clearer picture of what to expect if it is necessary to see a mental health professional.

Keeping diabetes in control is a delicate balancing act in which the factors that can increase blood glucose (eating, psychological stress, and infections) must be balanced against those that lower it (insulin and exercise). But there are also many ways in which effective coping with diabetes requires you to strike a delicate balance between competing psychological goals. You must balance your desire for your child to maintain normal blood glucose levels with your desire to raise children who have a strong personal identity apart from their diabetes. You must preserve your child's safety while promoting his or her independence. You must keep an eye on the future without neglecting the here and now. All of these difficult balancing acts are why I've written this book.

Since the publication of the first edition of this book 7 years ago, we've increased our understanding of what it takes to strike that fine balance between achieving good control of diabetes and helping our children grow into well-balanced, self-assured adults. In this book, I have framed this gradual development in terms of 10 key tasks that are faced by families of children and adolescents with diabetes. The 10 chapters lay out these keys, describe why each is important, explain how effective families will cope with that key task, offer practical methods of improving the family's response to that challenge, and suggest how to determine when you may need additional professional help.

You should look at this book much as you might a cookbook. Like a good cookbook, this book contains lots of "recipes" that hopefully sound appealing to you, things you'd like to try. Some may click for you on your first attempt. Others may not work out exactly as planned the first time around, so you may need to take a step back and figure out what went wrong. There may be other suggestions that don't seem to suit your needs or tastes quite as well. Some of you may be adventurous enough to use my ideas to create unique strategies that fit your situation and needs more closely than my general suggestions can.

In many chapters, I describe the fundamental treatment methods that are commonly used by child psychologists and other mental health professionals in their clinical practices. I do this for two reasons. First, I think that most of you, if given guidance and appropriate advice, can solve many of the parenting problems that diabetes sometimes creates. It may also be possible for you to prevent other issues from ever becoming problems. Second, I realize that some of you may face hurdles that are too complicated or long-lasting to be solved simply by reading a book. There are times when parents should seek the assistance of a mental health professional. Learning more about what to expect can help you be a more effective consumer, feel more comfortable about looking for a qualified mental health professional, and be a more capable participant in family or child therapy.

$$* \quad * \quad * \quad * \quad *$$

Many of you are probably familiar with the Food Pyramid for making healthy nutritional choices. I've borrowed this concept and applied it to parenting children with diabetes by placing the 10 key family tasks in the Diabetes Pyramid (see page x). The most fundamental keys form the base of the pyramid and are the foundation for dealing successfully with the more sophisticated and complex tasks that appear higher on the pyramid. Families who deal effectively with the lower, more basic levels will have a solid foundation that will better prepare them for dealing with the remaining key tasks. Families who continue to struggle with the more basic key tasks may find that, without this kind of stable foundation, accomplishing the more specialized keys nearer the top of the pyramid will be much more difficult.

As you read the following chapters, examine how your family deals with each of the specific tasks. No doubt you will find examples of problems and coping methods that are familiar to you and your family. Before you start reading this book, I want you to know that you're not going to be dealing with all 10 keys at the same time and that very few families have trouble with all of them. Despite the fact that growing up with diabetes brings with it complex psychological issues, I don't want you to feel overwhelmed by the special responsibilities that you face as parents. Most families do an admirable job of handling these challenges without the help of a psychologist or psychiatrist. This book is intended to help you feel more comfortable in your role by preparing you a little better. For some, this book may alert you to larger problems that you have not yet resolved or even recognized; hopefully you will be encouraged to take action to solve them. Most parents, if given the proper information and advice, will make the right choices for their children. For those of you who have infants and very young children with diabetes, you may feel that many of the topics covered in the book are too far in the future for you to worry about now. However, every one of the keys that I've covered in the 10 chapters of this book has its root in the very earliest years of childhood. You need to understand that you can begin helping your child with the 10 keys long before it is obvious. Also, knowing what you are shooting for in the long run and what problems you are trying to prevent is a very important ingredient in helping your child grow up to be as healthy as possible, both physically and mentally. At various points in the book, I've included practical suggestions for many of the common challenges that come with raising babies, toddlers, and preschoolers with diabetes. But try to remember that this book is really more about the big picture of raising a healthy young adult than it is a "how-to" guide.

Although this book offers a great deal of practical advice, there is no way that it can specifically address every concern that might be raised by parents, teachers, and others who take care of youngsters with diabetes. After 23 years in this profession, I know that I have yet to see every possible response by children with diabetes and their families to the disease. However, I've tried to emphasize the more common responses to diabetes and have provided some general frameworks for coping with other issues that might arise. Instead of focusing on problems, I have organized this book around 10 broad tasks that families face as a result of having a child with diabetes. I am convinced that families who address these keys successfully will someday look back at their experiences and know that they made the most of a difficult situation.

Relating to
Health
Professionals

School Adjustment

Social Skills

Diabetes Problem Solving

Treatment Adherence

Managing Stress

Family Sharing of Diabetes Responsibilities

Family Communication

Emotional Coping

Diabetes Knowledge

THE DIABETES PYRAMID

ACKNOWLEDGMENTS

Without the inspiration, encouragement, and assistance of many wonderful people, neither the first nor second edition of this book would have become a reality, and I'd like to mention those who have played important roles.

First of all, I've been privileged to have a very special relationship with hundreds of families over the years. While I learned a lot from them about coping with childhood diabetes, I learned even more about what's truly important and lasting. I consider myself very lucky to be able to enjoy a career that has been so personally rewarding and fulfilling. I hope that this book helps more families like yours raise children who grow up happy, healthy, and fulfilled.

I'd also like to thank my professional colleagues in pediatric psychology (Drs. Barbara Anderson, Michael Harris, Jill Weissberg-Benchell, Peggy Greco, Alan Delamater, Lisa Buckloh, Daniel Cox, and David Marrero), endocrinology (Drs. Neil White, Nelly Mauras, Larry Fox, Robert Olney, and Priscila Gagliardi), and nursing (Karen Wilkinson, Michelle Sadler, and Pamela Bulley) for their wisdom and insights. I realize how fortunate I am to be able to combine my professional work with so many wonderful friendships. I hope that I have done an adequate job of expressing the many lessons that all of you have shared with me.

KEY
1

DIABETES KNOWLEDGE

Emma was diagnosed with type 1 diabetes when she was 12 years old after her parents took her to a local urgent care center. She and her parents were taught how to do insulin injections and blood glucose tests, and they were given a pamphlet that included a sample diet. Other than that, they had no formal teaching about what diabetes is, what causes it, or why keeping blood glucose near normal levels is important. Afterward, a lot of people Emma knew told her stories about other people with diabetes, and many of these stories were very upsetting to her.

Emma gradually became discouraged and less and less careful about her diabetes responsibilities. About a year later, she was hospitalized because of very poor diabetes control, and while there, she told her doctor that she had been skipping her insulin injections a few times a week because she just couldn't make herself do it like she should. Emma's doctor referred her family to a diabetes educator and a dietitian to make sure they understood diabetes and its treatment. And since Emma was struggling with taking good care of herself, her doctor also referred her to a psychologist.

During her hospitalization, the team learned that Emma had many false beliefs about diabetes that were overwhelming to her. The doctor, nurse, dietitian, and psychologist worked as a team with Emma and her parents. As she learned more about diabetes, Emma gradually became more optimistic about her future and she began taking better care of herself. She was not hospitalized again.

KEY

1

DIABETES KNOWLEDGE

Diabetes knowledge belongs at the base of the Diabetes Pyramid because it is a must for everything that is to follow. Without accurate and up-to-date information about diabetes, every following task is made that much more difficult. But, if you and your child start off with a solid grasp of the basics and go on from there to become skilled diabetes self-managers, the other key tasks just seem to get done more smoothly and with less effort. There are a few key points about diabetes knowledge that every family needs to understand. Before getting on with these points, though, let's make sure that we're all consistent about the basic medical facts regarding diabetes and its treatment.

What You Need to Know: Diabetes 101

A thorough working knowledge of diabetes and its treatment is essential for healthy living with the disease. This job naturally falls to you as the parent of a child with diabetes. The information here is just a basic review and can't take the place of a complete family education about the medical aspects of diabetes. You'll have to get that:

▲ By taking classes taught by diabetes educators, such as nurses, physicians, and dietitians

▲ By reading other books that are available about diabetes care (see the "Resources" section)

▲ From real-life experience with diabetes problem solving

However, this section can serve as a solid introduction to diabetes and its treatment for people such as teachers, coaches, grandparents, and day-care providers, who might be involved in caring for your child in other ways. Although the primary responsibility for managing diabetes will always belong to the immediate family, many other people have important roles to play in promoting a healthy adjustment to this disease by your child. Accurate knowledge about diabetes is a crucial starting point in making this work.

What Is Type 1 Diabetes?

Type 1 diabetes mellitus is a disease that results when the pancreas, an organ that lies behind the stomach, stops making a hormone called *insulin*. Insulin's main function is to help the body use a sugar called *glucose* for energy, growth, and healing. When no insulin is available, your child's body cannot use the energy from foods that are eaten. This results in a kind of starvation in the cells. There is food there, the cells in the body just can't use it. During starvation, the body tries to use its own tissues (usually stored fat) for energy. The by-product of this burning of tissues is a toxic substance known as *ketones*, which collect in the blood and urine. Having high blood glucose levels over a long period of time probably caused your child to experience extreme thirst, more drinking, and more frequent urination. In the weeks and months before your child's diabetes was diagnosed, you may have noticed a sharp increase in your child's eating, drinking, and urination. Despite this, your child may have lost a lot of weight and seemed to lack energy (since his or her body wasn't getting the glucose it usually used for energy).

Unfortunately, once the body stops making insulin, it will never make insulin again. Once type 1 diabetes occurs, it is permanent.

What Causes Type 1 Diabetes?

After many years of research, scientists agree that type 1 diabetes is an *auto-immune* disease. This means that the body has reacted to some of its own tissue as if it were a foreign invader, like a virus or bacteria. In the case of type 1 diabetes, the body's immune defenses attack and destroy the *islet cells* in the pancreas that produce insulin (also known as beta cells). This occurs gradually, and the production of insulin ends gradually. The development of diabetes may take anywhere from several months to several years. Although scientists are getting closer to figuring out exactly why and how this happens, many questions remain.

The tendency to develop this kind of diabetes is partially genetic, but that is not the whole story. If your identical twin has type 1 diabetes, you have about a 30% to 50% chance of developing it yourself. If developing diabetes was determined totally by the genes parents pass onto their children, this chance would be 100% (since identical twins have identical genes).

Type 1 diabetes usually strikes during middle childhood, peaking among children at about 9 to 11 years old, but it can occur at any age. Research is being conducted to see whether it is possible to prevent this type of diabetes in relatives of people who already have it. Unfortunately, there is nothing that anyone could have done to keep it from happening to your child, and at this point, there is no way to reverse type 1 diabetes once it has developed.

How Is Type 1 Diabetes Treated?

Insulin

Right now, children and adolescents with type 1 diabetes must replace their natural levels of insulin daily. This can be done either by taking injections of insulin or by using the increasingly popular insulin pump, which is a small machine that constantly delivers a small amount of insulin, and larger doses of insulin before meals, through a small tube or needle that remains under the skin. In a later chapter (Key #7: Diabetes Problem Solving), I talk about the issues involved in deciding whether or not to use technological advances, such as insulin pumps, in your child's treatment. Many youngsters still take several insulin injections each day, usually just before meals and perhaps at bedtime. It is common for patients to take a mixture of two types of insulin that vary in how quickly they act and how long they last. Some youngsters may use the carbo-hydrate counting method, in which the amount of insulin given in each injection is based on the result of a blood glucose test done just before the injection and for the amount of carbohydrate they expect to eat.

Glucose testing
Insulin will have different effects on blood glucose levels in different children and from day to day in the same child. To recognize, and hopefully correct, unusually high or low blood glucose levels, people with diabetes are expected to test their blood glucose level several times each day. A common modern approach is to expect patients to test before meals (referred to as *pre-prandial*) and before bedtime, and to test now and then about 90 minutes after meals (*post-prandial*). A blood glucose test requires a drop of blood, either from the finger or from the thigh or forearm, depending on the glucose meter. The blood is placed on a strip and the strip is then placed into a blood glucose meter, which reads out the result and may store the test result in memory. Most diabetes health care teams and families prefer to also record the results in a logbook. A logbook of glucose readings provides a visual record that can make it easier to spot trends and solve problems. The test results should be used by fami-lies and by the health care team to make sure that the amount of insulin matches the child's eating habits and activities, with the goal of keeping the blood glucose level as normal as possible.

At clinic visits, a blood sample is usually obtained for an *A1C test* (also called glycohemoglobin, hemoglobin A_{1C}, or HbA_{1C}), which gives an estimate of average blood glucose levels over the past two to three months. There are several different methods of doing this test, so results from one clinic or laboratory cannot necessarily be com-pared directly to those done somewhere else. Your child's doctor can give you an idea of the levels that are viewed as excellent, fair, and poor diabetes control at your diabetes clinic.

Diet

Food and eating habits are also important parts of treating diabetes. Watching carbohydrates is especially important, since carbohydrates make up almost all of the glucose in the blood. In the past, the cornerstone of the diabetes diet was to avoid eating sugar. Doctors and nurses used to believe that eating sweets and sugar caused blood glucose levels to rise quicker than eating the same amount of carbohydrates from healthier food groups. We now know that this isn't true. The carbohydrates in an ice cream cone affect blood glucose levels the same way as the carbohydrates in potatoes, apples, rice, or broccoli. The modern approach to nutrition for children and adolescents with diabetes is to aim for a "constant-carbohydrate, low-fat" eating plan, often by teaching the child and parents how to count the amount of carbohydrate to be eaten at each meal. This places the emphasis more on consistency of eating habits, choosing healthy foods, and fitting the foods to the child's food preferences and habits, as opposed to the old way of simply avoiding refined sweets. Of course, candy and other sweets should still only be eaten every once in a while. Sweets contain lots of calories and not much else, so it is best for everyone to avoid concentrated sweets and to eat foods that are healthier and have more nutrients. Meals that are low in fat and include moderate amounts of protein may reduce the chances of certain long-term health problems that people with diabetes may develop. The bottom line? The healthiest diet for a child with diabetes is the diet that's healthy for everybody, with just a little more emphasis on steady levels of carbohydrates. If the diet helps maintain glucose levels and weight levels, the specific foods that are eaten are less important.

Exercise

Active exercise is an important part of every healthy child's day, and it is particularly important for children with diabetes. Since exercise helps to lower blood glucose levels, regular exercise can help people with diabetes get by with lower doses of insulin and allows them to eat more food. It also helps make the heart strong and healthy. Adults with diabetes are two to four times more susceptible to heart disease, so developing a lifestyle that includes regular exercise is even more important for youngsters with diabetes than it is for other children. Aerobic activities, such as running, swimming, cycling, tennis, and basketball, exert large muscles and make the heart and lungs work harder. These are the best kinds of exercise for people with diabetes. Although team sports, such as football, soccer, and baseball, are also good, these aren't activities that youngsters will be able to do for the rest of their lives.

Ups and downs

It's important for you to realize that, although treatment for diabetes is effective, it is still crude compared with how the body normally balances blood glucose levels and insulin production. Normally, the beta cells in the pancreas read the blood glucose level constantly and react very quickly to ups and downs by either increasing or decreasing the amount of insulin that is being released into the blood. People with diabetes have lost both of these basic functions. Modern treatment for diabetes substitutes blood glucose tests, perhaps four times a day, and several insulin injections for these natural processes. This is really a crude imitation of what the pancreas was designed to do, but it works. We are fortunate that there is an effective treatment for diabetes, but it also isn't too surprising that the treatment isn't always perfectly effective or 100% predictable.

The effects of insulin, food, and exercise on blood glucose levels vary from day to day. Every child or adolescent with diabetes will experience periods of very high blood glucose *(hyper*glycemia; blood glucose above 120–140 mg/dl) and abnormally low blood glucose *(hypo*glycemia; blood glucose below 60–70 mg/dl) that must be recognized and corrected. It's important to try to avoid severe highs and lows in blood glucose levels. Using blood glucose test results for problem solving can help children and their families predict and prevent highs and lows. Recognizing patterns in your child's glucose levels can help you develop an eating and insulin regimen that offers good control of your child's diabetes.

Hyperglycemia usually happens when not enough insulin has been taken or too much food has been eaten. Psychological stress and infections can also cause the blood glucose level to rise. Long-lasting hyperglycemia causes frequent drinking and urination, fatigue, and weight loss, just like when your child's diabetes was first detected. Very high blood glucose over a long period of time can lead to a condition known as *diabetic ketoacidosis*, an emergency situation that requires hospitalization.

Hypoglycemia usually happens because not enough food has been eaten, activity levels were too high, or too much insulin was given. Sometimes hypoglycemia happens several hours after an intense period of activity. Symptoms of low blood glucose may include dizziness, sweating, trembling, and confusion. Low blood glucose reactions, also known as insulin reactions, must be stopped from getting worse by eating or drinking something containing sugar. If allowed to become severe, hypoglycemia can result in loss of consciousness or seizures (like those that happen to people with epilepsy), and your child may require an injection of glucagon, a hormone that raises the blood glucose level very quickly. Because a child's central nervous system is still developing and maturing, most doctors try to keep severe hypoglycemia to a bare minimum. When your child has a low blood sugar, hormones are released that cause the liver to release stored glucose into the blood stream, resulting in an increase in blood sugar. Many of the obvious symptoms of hypoglycemia (sweating, trembling, nausea) are due to these hormones. Having frequent mild hypoglycemia can cause your child's body to use up its stores of these hormones, resulting in your child's loss of the body's normal signals and cues that indicate a low blood sugar (sometimes known as *hypoglycemia insensitivity*). This can result in episodes of severe hypoglycemia that can progress to seizures, fainting, and an inability to correct the low blood sugar without help from someone else. So, if your child has several low blood sugars in a short period of time, you and you child need to be really careful in order to prevent more severe hypoglycemia.

What Is Type 2 Diabetes?

The far more common form of diabetes among all age groups is type 2 diabetes. Type 2 diabetes affects over 90% of all people with diabetes, and there are probably many people who have the disease who don't know it. Although type 2 diabetes used to occur almost entirely in middle-aged and older adults, it has become more and more common among kids, especially in Hispanic and African-American minorities.

Unlike type 1 diabetes, which is caused when the body stops making insulin altogether, type 2 diabetes in youth begins with a period of increasing insulin resistance, in which the body loses its sensitivity to the insulin that the pancreas is producing. This insensitivity to insulin causes the pancreas to secrete larger and larger amounts of insulin as the body tries harder and harder to get glucose levels back to normal. During these early stages of type 2 diabetes, it is often possible to treat the condition with diet and exercise alone. Other patients may need oral medications that reduce glucose levels or increase the body's sensitivity to insulin. Unfortunately, in most children and adolescents with type 2 diabetes the cells in the pancreas that make insulin eventually wear out and stop producing insulin altogether. Once the disease reaches that stage, treatment is essentially the same as that for type 1 diabetes.

What Causes Type 2 Diabetes?

The best way to answer this question is to say that the tendency to develop type 2 diabetes is definitely inherited, and a lifestyle consisting of overeating and little physical exercise makes it much more likely that this tendency will be fulfilled. So, the causes of type 2 diabetes that we can control are the very same habits that have become so deeply ingrained in our culture: fast food, super-sizing, eating while watching TV, spending hours on the internet or playing video games, riding cars or buses, and generally being couch potatoes. Therefore, if you have a child who has developed type 2 diabetes, any other children you have may be at risk of developing the disease too. But, you can help prevent this by encouraging your other children to lose weight, exercise more regularly, and adopt healthier eating habits for the rest of their lives. The challenges faced by parents in accomplishing these difficult goals are the topic of several sections to come later in this book.

What About Long-Term Health Problems?

I was once sitting in a hospital room with an 11-year-old boy who had been diagnosed with type 1 diabetes about two days earlier when the TV set in his room showed a commercial by the American Diabetes Association. The commercial encouraged people to give money to fight diabetes, a leading cause of blindness. I realized then that not very many kids with recently diagnosed diabetes are fortunate enough to have a child psychologist sitting next to them when they first encounter this kind of news. Since then, I have learned that it is common for children, and their parents, to be told various extremely scary stories about the dire long-term effects of diabetes, some often wrong, by friends, relatives, and neighbors. Many health care professionals prefer to avoid burdening children and their parents with information about diabetes complications in the beginning. This may be because diabetes complications are rare until adulthood or because there is a lot of information about diabetes complications, much of it very complex. On the other hand, many parents have told me that they would have preferred to have received detailed, accurate information about diabetes complications at or near the time of diagnosis. Having this information "concealed" from them only made them wonder why they hadn't been told, led them to think the situation was even worse than it is, and caused some to lose trust in their doctors and nurses from the beginning.

So, there is little to be gained by withholding the straight facts. People with diabetes do face increased risks of several serious health problems, but usually only after years of high blood glucose levels. Unfortunately, individuals in racial and ethnic minorities are more likely to develop these problems than are whites, and it is unclear whether this is due to differences in the quality of or access to health care, self-management behaviors, or genetic tendencies. These health problems can include damage to very tiny blood vessels (*microvascular problems*), large blood vessels (*macrovascular problems*), and nerves (*neuropathy*).

Microvascular problems can affect many different organs, including the eyes, resulting in possible loss of vision (*retinopathy*), and the kidneys, resulting in possible kidney damage (*nephropathy*).

Macrovascular problems affect the heart and circulation and are the reason diabetes is a major risk factor for heart attacks and other circulation problems, such as stroke. Nerve damage can result in loss of sensation or feelings of tingling, burning, or pain, commonly in the feet and legs, or disruption of basic body functions, such as digestion and control of heart rate. Also, women with diabetes must be very careful to maintain excellent blood glucose control before and throughout pregnancy, which can prevent serious medical problems in developing babies. There is no reason women with diabetes should avoid pregnancy if they are generally in good health, each pregnancy is planned, and they are careful about meeting tight blood glucose goals before and throughout the pregnancy.

The outlook for the long-term health of people with diabetes is not all gloom and doom. Thanks to a large-scale study called the Diabetes Control and Complications Trial (DCCT), there is now proof that maintaining near-normal blood glucose levels greatly delays the onset and slows the progress of the complications of diabetes. At 29 treatment centers around North America, 1,441 patients with type 1 diabetes were assigned randomly to either conventional diabetes therapy or intensive therapy. Intensive therapy included more frequent clinical visits, more frequent insulin injections and blood glucose tests, telephone contact with a diabetes nurse at least once a week, and help from dietitians and psychologists, all with a goal of keeping blood glucose levels as close to normal as possible. The conventional therapy patients maintained their standard diabetes care routines, which included fewer insulin injections and blood glucose tests each day, and less emphasis on keeping their blood glucose levels close to normal compared with the intensive therapy group. The patients were followed for about 7 years, and the onset and progress of diabetes complications were measured regularly. As expected, the intensive therapy group was in much better diabetic control than the conventional therapy group throughout the study.

The fact is that, even with all of the extra support available to them, only about 5% of the DCCT intensive therapy patients maintained near-normal blood glucose levels consistently. Even fewer of the teenagers in the study did so. But despite less-than-perfect glucose control, the intensive therapy patients had a 50% to 75%

reduction in eye, kidney, and nerve problems, compared with patients treated with conventional therapy. It wasn't necessary to achieve perfect glucose control, because *any* sustained reduction in blood sugars reduced the onset and progression of long-term complications. The main message to be taken from these results is that the scary long-term complications of diabetes aren't completely beyond the control of people with diabetes and their families.

Our research team has completed a similar evaluation of intensive therapy for 6- to 15-year-old children with type 1 diabetes, except that our goal was to determine if this approach is safe and effective in achieving better diabetic control in pediatric patients. We found that, compared with usual medical care, children treated with intensive therapy had better diabetic control, with no increase in either severe hypoglycemia or unwanted weight gain. Intensive therapy was beneficial for children across the board, regardless of race, ethnicity, socioeconomic status, and diabetes self-management skills when they entered the study.

A similar long-term British study, called the United Kingdom Prospective Diabetes Study (UKPDS), was done with adults who had type 2 diabetes. Again, keeping blood sugars near normal over a period of years greatly reduced both the onset and the progression of diabetes complications. So the DCCT findings seemed to hold for type 2 diabetes as well.

Realistically, these threats of long-term health problems can be reduced greatly by keeping diabetes in good control over the long haul. The DCCT and UKPDS also showed that our available medical tools are suited to accomplishing this, and it taught health care professionals many valuable lessons about how to help their patients achieve and maintain better diabetes control. As more advances are made in insulin, glucose meters, insulin delivery devices, and continuous glucose sensors, and as more varied and flexible treatment regimens are tested and refined, excellent diabetic control should be more easily achieved than in the past. Many effective tools exist now to help you, your child, and your health care team work together to keep your child in the best possible health for as long as possible.

Overall, there are several good reasons why a person who develops diabetes today should feel less threatened by the risk of long-term complications than people who have had the disease a lot longer. Recognition of the long-term complications of diabetes didn't even begin to surface widely until the 1950s and 1960s. Only recently has careful research absolutely proven that glucose control affects whether or not complications develop. Before the DCCT and UKPDS, many doctors who cared for children with diabetes weren't convinced of the need for youngsters to strive for tight glucose control. The American Diabetes Association's *Clinical Practice Recommendations* states that keeping blood glucose as close to normal as possible should be the goal for all patients with diabetes unless there are special extenuating circumstances (such as for very young children who may be at increased risk of severe hypoglycemia. Striving for near-normal blood glucose is generally considered less advisable for them). There have been constant improvements in our ability to detect diabetes complications early and it is usually true in medicine that the earlier a problem is found, the more options exist for correcting it. Also, methods of treating the complications have improved steadily, and this will probably continue. Finally, diabetes is such a common disease that the government, industry, and organizations like the American Diabetes Association continue to devote huge amounts of money to research projects that have an excellent chance of leading to better methods of detecting and treating the complications. Later in this book, I give advice about how to talk with your child about the sensitive topic of diabetes complications. I believe that if the subject of long-term complications is dealt with properly, it can go a long way toward maintaining a productive health partnership with your child throughout adolescence.

Will Diabetes Ever Be Cured?

The beta cells in your child's pancreas will never start producing insulin again, but there are diabetes treatments on the horizon that come very close to what could be called a "cure". Pancreas transplantation has been done for many years. However, this procedure is generally reserved for people with very poor health due to advanced long-term complications of diabetes, usually people who need a kidney transplant and who will be taking anti-rejection drugs anyway. And there aren't nearly enough pancreas donors to make this a workable option for all people with diabetes, so other avenues are being explored. One of these is the transplantation of only the insulin-producing portion of the pancreas—the beta, or islet, cells. Another approach is the development of an artificial pancreas. This might take the form of an implanted glucose sensor that gives immediate and continuous feedback about blood glucose levels to a device like an insulin pump, which regulates how much insulin to give. This approach currently faces some significant technical problems, but a great deal of work is going on to overcome these obstacles. There are already several FDA-approved devices that can be called "continuous glucose sensors" and others are in development. The available devices track glucose levels in the fluid between cells and estimate blood glucose levels based on this information. Presently, these devices aren't accurate enough to replace regular blood sugar tests, but that may eventually be a possibility. The day may come when finger-stick blood glucose tests will be a thing of the past.

Although it would be a little foolish to believe that these approaches will lead quickly to something resembling a cure for diabetes, it would perhaps be even more foolish to think that the future holds no promise for people with diabetes. At the very least one can say with some certainty that future advances will provide more and better treatment alternatives for people with diabetes than we have now.

Why Diabetes Knowledge Is Critical

The old saying "knowledge is power" is never truer than when it comes to diabetes. First, the more you and your family understand about diabetes, the better off physically your child with diabetes will be. There is probably no medical condition that places more treatment responsibility on the patient and family than diabetes. Whether you want to accept this role or not, you and your child are the captains of your child's health care team. You must understand the how, what, why, and when of diabetes management in order to be effective in that role. Second, the advantages of diabetes knowledge extend to the emotional health of your child and family as well. Understanding clearly what you are up against, and what tools and resources you have to help you deal with those challenges, is a key ingredient in helping you and your child to cope with the emotional pain that diabetes can cause.

Diabetes Knowledge Aids Emotional Coping

Regardless of the circumstances of your child's diagnosis, every member of the family must deal with the shock, pain, and fear that comes with this bad news in his or her own way. Learning that diabetes is controllable, recognizing that it wasn't caused by anything that could have been anticipated or prevented, understanding the specific tasks required in its treatment, and achieving rapid success in acquiring the skills needed to accomplish those tasks can all play important roles in the process of emotional heating. On the other hand, inadequate knowledge about diabetes is often at the core of those lingering emotional sore spots that many people with diabetes seem to endure. As the remaining chapters of this book show, there are plenty of factors other than diabetes knowledge that affect people's emotional adjustment to the disease, but learning about diabetes and constantly expanding your knowledge are two of the most important tools you have available to help you stay on top of the emotional side of diabetes.

Diabetes Knowledge Protects Against Misinformation

There are many good sources of accurate information about diabetes available to anyone who wants to find it. But, there are also a lot of myths and misconceptions about diabetes out there, and you and your child need to be able to recognize them. Diabetes is such a common disease that most people know someone with either type 1 or type 2 diabetes. So, there is a good chance that one or more members of your family, or some of your neighbors or co-workers, have preconceived ideas about diabetes that they may share with you or your child. After the diagnosis, friends, neighbors, relatives, co-workers, and classmates may tell you their own stories about their personal experiences with diabetes, and these may or may not be accurate. Many of these stories, even though they are usually offered in a sharing and supportive spirit, may be based on false, incomplete, or outdated information about diabetes.

Diabetes intrudes into just about every aspect of a child's daily life, including eating, school, travel, and sports. As a result, families and children with diabetes will have to interact frequently with many people who have little or no understanding of diabetes. For all of these reasons, arming yourself with accurate, up-to-date information about diabetes and its treatment is the best way to protect you and your child from these potential trouble spots.

Survival Skills Education

If I were asked to design an educational situation that makes it as hard as possible to learn important facts and skills, I don't think I could do a better job than the circumstances that face most newly diagnosed patients and their families. Your normal family routines of eating, working, and going to school were interrupted, and your child was also removed from his or her comfortable surroundings and put into a hospital setting with other seriously ill children. Some may even have spent some time in an intensive care unit. Family members often experience all kinds of intense emotions like anxiety, guilt, confusion, fear, and self-doubt. You and your child may have been deprived of sleep and perhaps separated from the rest of the family. At the same time, you were all placed under considerable pressure to learn a great deal of technical information and skills and perhaps forced to overcome a lifelong fear of injections and blood. When you look at it this way, I'm surprised that so many families do such a great job of acquiring the basic diabetes knowledge and skills they need to use right away, the so-called survival skills of diabetes, so quickly and effectively. Luckily, the very process of diabetes education helps to lower some of these obstacles, and most children and their families begin their emotional recovery quickly after their diagnosis.

Diabetes Knowledge "Checkups"

Every youngster with diabetes needs periodic medical checkups to keep track of special health problems. For a number of reasons, it's also important that a diabetes educator regularly reevaluate your diabetes knowledge and skills, and your child's, so that your skills can be refined and updated. Gaining new knowledge about diabetes and keeping your diabetes skills sharp are two important aspects of diabetes care. Many published studies of nurses, laboratory technicians, and other medical personnel show that technical skills and knowledge tend to drop off over time, particularly for tasks and concepts that aren't used very often. When any task is done repeatedly, people tend to drift into their own unique way of performing the skill if their technique isn't examined and refined periodically. This is also true of children with diabetes and their parents. For example, one study found that mothers and fathers of children with diabetes differed significantly in the accuracy with which they drew up prescribed insulin doses. This means that, if the parents sometimes traded off the responsibility for drawing up their children's insulin doses, the actual amount of insulin that the child received would vary depending on which parent was giving the injection. Other studies have shown that accuracy in estimating food portions by children with diabetes and their parents drops over time and that errors in blood glucose testing increase over time. This shows how important it is to check the skills of everyone involved in your child's diabetes care now and then, compare them to what you were taught, and refine them as needed.

Another good reason for continuing your diabetes education and getting periodic diabetes knowledge "checkups" is that diabetes self-management methods are constantly evolving as new products are made available and previous methods are refined and improved. I'm sure you'd want to use any advances available to your child as soon as you can.

Evaluating Your Diabetes Education Program

Many hospitals, clinics, physicians, and private consultants offer diabetes education services. For a number of years, the American Diabetes Association has officially recognized diabetes patient education programs that meet national standards based on their structure, content, and quality. (To find an education program in your area that has achieved recognition, see the Resources section.) If there isn't a recognized program that's convenient for you, it's important that you know how to evaluate the diabetes education services that are available to you. Here are some important questions to ask regarding the structure of a program:

▲ Do the instructors have current qualifications as Certified Diabetes Educators (CDE) from the American Association of Diabetes Educators?

▲ Does the program staff include a nurse and dietitian?

▲ Does the program have extensive experience working with children and adolescents and their families?

▲ Does the program have an established working relationship with your child's physician?

▲ Does the program use educational materials that are specifically designed for children and adolescents with diabetes and their families?

▲ Have any members of the program staff received recent continuing education credits on topics concerning children with diabetes?

In addition to these features, it is also important that your education focus on certain areas. Programs recognized by the American Diabetes Association are required to offer up-to-date instruction on these 15 aspects of diabetes and its treatment:

1. Diabetes overview

2. Stress and psychosocial adjustment

3. Family involvement and social support

4. Nutrition

5. Exercise and activity

6. Medications

7. Monitoring and use of results

8. Relationships between nutrition, exercise, medication, and blood glucose levels

9. Prevention, detection, and treatment of acute complications

10. Prevention, detection, and treatment of chronic complications

11. Foot, skin, and dental care

12. Behavior-change strategies, goal setting, risk-factor reduction, and problem solving

13. Benefits, risks, and management options for improving glucose control

14. Preconception care, pregnancy, and gestational diabetes

15. Use of health care systems and community resources

Going Beyond the Classroom

An important purpose of diabetes education in the beginning is to help families become lifelong students of diabetes by showing them how important diabetes knowledge really is. There are countless ways to improve and expand your knowledge of diabetes outside of structured classes. I've included detailed information in Resources about how to take advantage of opportunities, such as these:

▲ Arrange for your child to attend a diabetes summer camp or other diabetes-related recreational program.

▲ Subscribe to and read magazines, such as Diabetes Forecast.

▲ Become active in local or statewide chapters of the American Diabetes Association.

▲ Attend, or start, an educational diabetes support group for patients, family members, and youngsters with diabetes.

▲ Take advantage of on-line diabetes information and services.

▲ Read books about childhood diabetes.

Becoming an Expert on Your Child's Diabetes

I suppose the overall goal of modern diabetes treatment is to help your child become an independently functioning young adult who handles the typical hurdles and challenges that life has to offer while coping effectively with the special demands of diabetes. If you want to help your child achieve that level of healthy independence, it makes sense to help your child become an expert on his or her diabetes as early as possible.

Diabetes is almost a different disease in every child that it strikes. Although the basic principles of diabetes and diabetes care are the same, every family, child, personality type, and individual body reacts to diabetes in subtle, unique, and complex ways. I can't tell you how your child is special, but I can tell you that every child's physical and emotional responses to diabetes are unique in some way. Discovering these special features, and putting them to work for you and your child, is an important continuing goal of diabetes education. For example, I once spoke with a mother who had some pretty convincing evidence that taking a shower caused her daughter's blood glucose level to drop sharply by as much as 100 to 150 mg/dl. I couldn't give her a reasonable physiological explanation about why this would happen, but I'm not sure that was really necessary anyway. Just knowing that her daughter's blood glucose was affected fairly consistently by the hot water prepared the mother to help her daughter avoid low blood glucose reactions. Plus, she had another tool to use when her daughter's blood glucose was too high. This mother and daughter illustrated for me that the more you know about diabetes, the easier it will be for you and your child to become experts on the unique aspects of your child's diabetes, helping your child gain the confidence needed to really take charge of living with diabetes as a young adult.

For Fathers Only

For about 90% of all children and adolescents with diabetes, mothers assume the primary responsibility for monitoring the child's diabetes, dealing with medical appointments, keeping track of supplies, and making sure that the child sticks with the demands of diabetes treatment. There are many reasons why this might be the case and there are many families in which this arrangement works well. Other families, though, have found that when parents share the burdens posed by diabetes, things simply go better for everyone involved. Sure, there are many practical barriers that can prevent some fathers from being as actively involved in the child's diabetes care as they might prefer. But, learning about diabetes and its treatment can be done on your own schedule and at your own pace. Learning about diabetes and refining your knowledge afterwards can bring you several kinds of benefits:

▲ Your partner will feel less isolated and more supported in taking on the huge responsibilities that come with managing diabetes.

▲ Your child will see you as being interested in and committed to a very important aspect of his or her life.

▲ You will be better prepared to solve diabetes-related problems that your child may experience rather than feeling helpless or, worse yet, making a mistake.

▲ Your family will have less friction and fewer diabetes-related hassles because everyone will be on the same page.

So, for all of these reasons, I think fathers should learn as much as they can about their children's diabetes. If you happen to be a father who doesn't have custody, I think you have even more to gain by doing so. The Resources section at the end of this book gives you many ways to acquire and refine your diabetes knowledge. Or, you can contact your child's diabetes doctor for information about local diabetes education programs.

Why Knowledge Alone Isn't Enough

On the surface, people seem to be rational creatures who, if given the correct and necessary information, usually make the right decisions with their lives. But there is a lot of scientific data suggesting that people, especially children and adolescents, do not necessarily behave rationally or logically, particularly when it comes to health-related behaviors. For instance, many people continue to drive without wearing seat belts or smoke cigarettes despite the possible health consequences of these behaviors. Although knowledge about diabetes is the most important first step in coping with all of the other tasks posed by living with diabetes, having sound knowledge about diabetes by itself doesn't guarantee good emotional adjustment to the disease, good cooperation in self-care responsibilities, or near-normal blood glucose control. Things are much more complicated than that. If just knowing about diabetes and its treatment were enough, everyone with adequate diabetes knowledge would be in perfect diabetic control. But, as your diabetes educator can tell you, knowledge alone isn't enough. In fact, quite a few studies have shown that diabetes knowledge by itself is not a very strong predictor of blood glucose control. The tasks of achieving and maintaining near-normal blood glucose levels are immensely more complicated than simply having adequate knowledge of diabetes concepts and skills. Although accurate knowledge about diabetes is required to achieve blood glucose goals, many other factors affect whether this knowledge can be used effectively to reach those goals. Diabetes deals out some wild cards, like your child's unique metabolism and psychological makeup. Knowledge alone doesn't guarantee that emotional adaptation will necessarily proceed smoothly. Learning how to put your diabetes knowledge to work to achieve good control of diabetes while promoting your child's mental health is the rest of the challenge.

TAKE-HOME MESSAGE

1

Effective parenting of youngsters with diabetes must be based on a solid foundation of accurate knowledge about diabetes and its treatment. Your base of knowledge should be refined and updated constantly so that you can become an expert on your child's diabetes.

K E Y
2

EMOTIONAL COPING

Diabetes Knowledge

Justin was a 17-year-old high school swimmer whose diabetes was detected when he was getting a physical exam for school sports. During his hospital stay after being first diagnosed, he had major emotional reactions to the injections and finger-sticks and he had a very hard time accepting that he had to learn these skills. Several times during teaching sessions, he broke down crying and had to leave the room. Before all of this happened, Justin was a very good student, and his parents said that he was extremely well-behaved and cooperative.

Teaching Justin about diabetes wasn't enough to help him get over the emotional shock and pain that came with the diagnosis. After going home from the hospital, Justin's mother called the clinic several times, worried about his severe emotional outbursts when it was time for shots or tests. Justin was referred to a psychologist for counseling, and he also took part in a support group for teenagers with diabetes. Eventually he learned to cope with his diabetes and returned to competitive swimming, earning a college scholarship.

KEY

2

EMOTIONAL COPING

Diabetes hurts! When you received the news that your child had diabetes, many of your first thoughts (and those of your child) probably centered on the physical pain that goes along with insulin injections and blood glucose tests. But diabetes also hurts *emotionally,* and until some of this emotional pain heals, it's often difficult for parents or youngsters with diabetes to turn their attention and energy toward the remaining tasks.

Just about every child with diabetes feels emotional pain when he or she is diagnosed. This pain is likely to resurface later, too, at times when diabetes makes it hard to just be a kid. As a result, the children who continue to suffer the greatest emotional pain from having diabetes often have the most trouble taking care of themselves and controlling their diabetes. This only further fuels their anger, fear, and resentment, and can result in even more deeply rooted and lasting emotional turmoil.

I know you don't want your child's diabetes to be unnecessarily painful, disabling, or burdensome, so it's important to understand the natural emotional reactions to diabetes and to have some sense of how to help your child deal with these reactions. You should expect your child to have emotional low points concerning diabetes and prepare yourself for these times. Many parents are terribly uncomfortable about this because there seems to be absolutely nothing they can do to ease their child's suffering. But there are two very helpful things that you can do. First, try your best to create an emotionally supportive family environment to reduce the frequency and intensity of the emotional storms that do arise (we'll talk more about this later). Second, learn how to react correctly when your child hits an emotional low. This is a challenging aspect of raising a child with diabetes, but dealing successfully with this task really lowers many of the other hurdles that you and your child will face in coping with diabetes.

Knowing as much as you can about the physical part of diabetes plays a big part in helping your family cope with the emotional side of having diabetes. Learning about diabetes will remove or reduce any feelings of guilt that you may have about your child's diabetes. It will help you cope with anxiety about long-term complications. Education also paves the way for youngsters to overcome their initial fears and worries about having this disease. But gaining or refining knowledge is not enough to help every parent and child deal with some of their complex feelings.

Because diabetes shows up in nearly every aspect of daily life, carrying around excess emotional baggage can really make life tough for kids with diabetes, parents, and even other family members. I like to recommend that, while taking diabetes seriously and being careful about blood glucose levels, you attempt to give diabetes care a minimum share of your time and energy. As you can imagine, this is nearly impossible if treatment responsibilities stir up negative feelings like anger, guilt, resentment, burnout, and fear. Everyone has these feelings at times. The key is learning how to get through these feelings without letting them keep you, or your child, down for too long. In this chapter, I describe some of the common negative emotional responses to diabetes and give some suggestions on how they can be prevented, reduced, or corrected.

What Are We Striving For?

When you're hoping to make changes, it's helpful to have a goal or an ideal to shoot for. Here are some examples of healthy emotional adjustments to diabetes and what factors promote them. Remember that healthy emotional adjustment to diabetes is a process, not a single event. It's a long-term effort to keep on top of the emotional challenges that diabetes creates and to stay positive despite occasional setbacks and disappointments. When youngsters with diabetes (and their parents) have achieved a healthy emotional adjustment to diabetes, they're likely to have some (but not necessarily all) of these characteristics:

▲ They view controlling diabetes as something broader than simply achieving a certain A1C level. Controlling diabetes means living a full and satisfying life and meeting personal goals despite diabetes.

▲ They feel successful in other parts of their lives, such as school, sports, friendships, or church, and don't let diabetes stand in the way of going after important goals.

▲ Diabetes occupies only a small part of their thoughts and energy during the day. Daily self-care activities become automatic habits that have about the same level of emotional significance as doing homework or completing household chores. Although they complete their self-care activities carefully, they view these tasks as necessary responsibilities for healthy living and not as a terrible burden.

▲ When necessary, they are able to tell others about their diabetes without feeling ashamed or embarrassed.

▲ They recover quickly from setbacks and disappointments regarding diabetes and view these as learning opportunities and challenges for the future rather than as a curse.

▲ People close to them respect them as heroes for dealing with diabetes without getting discouraged.

I have yet to meet a person with diabetes who has all of these characteristics all of the time. You and your child may want to set these ideals as goals to work toward, but don't expect to one day find that your work is finished. It's more realistic to think of healthy coping with diabetes as a process of striving toward goals that will be interrupted by setbacks and obstacles from time to time.

Learning to cope with troubles, barriers, and disappointments is a natural part of life for everyone, and people with diabetes are no exception. What's important is making sure that as you and your child work your way through this process, both of you receive something of value, such as worthwhile lessons, increased personal strength, or even a renewed commitment to try harder in the future. These are lofty standards to strive for, but any youngster with diabetes can work toward these ideals.

As important as it is to have goals, it's equally important to recognize the significant psychological challenges that diabetes poses to your child, to other children in the family, and to you. Although defining these challenges may seem a little gloomy, they are part of the reality of living with diabetes.

Common Emotional Pitfalls Among Children and Adolescents

No one gets to choose if or when he or she will get diabetes, and some kids are already psychologically vulnerable when diabetes enters their life. Youngsters who have had a life punctuated with other bad experiences or who have strong family histories of psychological disorders may be likely to have trouble coping with the emotional side of diabetes.

Despite the burden imposed by diabetes, there is still disagreement among behavioral scientists about whether kids with diabetes suffer more frequent or serious psychological and emotional disorders than kids without diabetes. However, it is clear that kids with diabetes who do suffer from emotional or psychological problems are much more likely to have poor glucose control.

Most youngsters go through a grieving process when they are newly diagnosed. The severity of this process varies tremendously from one child to the next. The reactions can range from fear of needles and lancets for young children, to adult-like depression in older adolescents. For most, it is a temporary reaction that doesn't interfere noticeably with their functioning once they've lived with diabetes for a few months. Emotional flare-ups may tend to surface during times when your child is facing other big hurdles, like starting class at a new school or beginning to date. However, some continue to suffer bouts of emotional turmoil, such as anger, resentment, denial of the severity of the disease, or a sense of unfairness, for years after diagnosis. Children who have had a succession of bad experiences in life, such as divorce, failure at school, peer rejection, or body image problems, run a greater risk for continued difficulty with the emotional adjustment to diabetes. This high-risk group should probably see a mental health professional at least as frequently as they see their doctors and nurses.

The first few months after diagnosis are crucial in setting the stage for a child's later adjustment to diabetes. Psychological treatments like support groups and group therapy for youngsters with diabetes may show the best results when they're offered just after diagnosis. It is also during these first few months of diabetes that youngsters may be most likely to express anger, resentment, and frustration about having diabetes. This makes most parents uncomfortable, because there really isn't anything that can be done to change or fix the situation. Your reaction may be to discourage these kinds of emotional expressions by dismissing or minimizing your child's concerns, changing the subject, or suggesting that he or she talk to someone else about it. However, the most helpful response that you can give when your child is agonizing about diabetes is simply to listen, sympathize, and let him or her know that these feelings are natural and understandable.

I have seen emotional reactions to diabetes among older children and adolescents that can make the condition much more disabling than it needs to be. For some youngsters, these reactions seem to be a chronic part of living with diabetes. For others, these responses surface mostly when they're having a tough time with life in general. It's common for the following reactions to be clustered together within the same child:

▲ Believing that all or most bad experiences are due to having diabetes, often accompanied by feelings of intense bitterness toward diabetes and everything associated with it

▲ Defining one's identity largely or primarily in terms of having diabetes

▲ Believing that people without diabetes cannot possibly relate to, or show compassion for, the experiences of a person with diabetes

▲ Insisting that better adjustment to diabetes is impossible and therefore cooperation with treatment is useless

▲ Avoiding interactions with others who have diabetes and refusal to acquire new information about diabetes

▲ Believing that diabetes carries with it many restrictions and limitations that deprive a person of a normal range of opportunities and alternatives

This kind of all-or-nothing thinking magnifies the negative aspects of diabetes well out of proportion to reality and can restrict and harm your child. These beliefs also tend to become self-fulfilling prophecies, causing youngsters with diabetes to close a lot of doors for themselves and to deprive themselves of normal opportunities and experiences.

There are many ways in which parents may inadvertently contribute to the development of these negative attitudes. The most common and important way is by overemphasizing diabetes as a cause of the youngster's thoughts, feelings, and actions. A childhood diabetes specialist, Dr. Luther Travis, encouraged using the term *child with diabetes* rather than *diabetic child* to emphasize the importance of treating the child as a unique individual who happens to carry along this thing called diabetes. Many older adolescents have told me that they really resented being viewed as a "diabetic" rather than as a person. The overemphasis of their blood glucose levels by their parents is one of the most common examples of this. By routinely interpreting every unusual behavior or emotion as first and foremost a sign of high or low blood glucose or simply by dwelling on the child's diabetes too much, parents may convince the child that diabetes is at the core of his or her identity. I have seen many adolescents with diabetes who deeply resented being viewed in this way by those close to them and who desperately wanted to be treated as individuals who happen to have diabetes. In fact, research hasn't really shown that moods are consistently correlated with blood glucose levels or that adolescents with diabetes and their parents can accurately estimate the child's blood glucose simply by the youngster's moods.

Other family environment factors that could over-emphasize the importance of diabetes in defining a youngster's identity include:

- Frequent negative interactions and criticism regarding the child's diabetes self-care without corresponding praise and acknowledgment for self-care successes
- Inference that diabetes is a form of punishment for sins or other misdeeds committed in the past
- Insufficient emotional support from parents and other family members and discomfort with discussing the emotional side of living with diabetes
- Allowing the child to avoid responsibilities frequently by being or acting sick
- Preferential treatment of the child with diabetes compared with brothers and sisters
- Infrequent or insufficient acknowledgment of the child's talents, skills, and accomplishments in other aspects of life

There are a few situations in which youngsters with diabetes may develop psychological disorders that require evaluation and treatment by a mental health professional. Prolonged or severe emotional difficulties surrounding diabetes may be part of an episode of depression, and this may be the most common psychological disorder among children and adolescents with diabetes. One long-term study showed that about a quarter of adolescents and young adults suffered depression during the first 10 years after they were diagnosed with type 1 diabetes. Among adolescents, the symptoms of depression can include:

- Feelings of low self-esteem
- Persistent sadness
- Guilt
- Thoughts about suicide

- ▲ Psychosomatic symptoms, such as headaches and abdominal pain
- ▲ Increases or decreases in sleep or appetite
- ▲ Poor school performance
- ▲ Reduced energy and initiative
- ▲ Withdrawal from friends or activities
- ▲ Poor concentration and memory

Depression can be treated very effectively with psychotherapy, anti-depressant medication, or a combination of the two. If your child shows most of these characteristics over a period of more than two to three months, or if there is any hint of suicidal thoughts, I recommend seeing a mental health professional to determine whether your child is depressed and to help your child recover emotionally.

Diabetes treatment puts a lot of emphasis on food and eating habits. Many children lose quite a bit of weight in the weeks and months just before being diagnosed with type 1 diabetes. Then, when they're started on insulin, much of the lost weight is regained. Youngsters who maintain excellent glucose control are also likely to experience weight gain. These factors may increase the risk of weight-related concerns and eating with diabetes, especially among young women. Many studies have looked at whether young women with diabetes are at an increased risk of eating disorders, such as anorexia nervosa (eating far too little) and bulimia (periodic binge-eating episodes, often followed by vomiting or other means of purging). These studies have yet to produce any clear conclusions, and it is still debated whether young women with diabetes are more likely than other women to have eating disorders. Nonetheless, young women who have eating disorders clearly run a high risk for poor diabetic control and repeated hospitalizations. Poor glucose control may also be due in part to an intentional under-treatment with insulin in an effort to lose weight. Give this possibility some thought if you have a youngster, especially a teenage girl, who shows wide swings in glucose control that you don't understand. Evidence of an eating disorder (such as a tendency for a kid to see herself as being overweight when she isn't or more overweight than she really is, to be driven to excel in school or sports, and to be afraid of the independence and responsibility that come with growing up) is another reason to seek out a mental health professional.

Some children with diabetes, especially those older than about seven, can develop an understandable fear of hypoglycemia. This may cause them to actively avoid having near-normal blood glucose and to keep their blood glucose constantly on the high side, leading to glucose control that is not close to the treatment goal. A fear of hypoglycemia may also be accompanied by premature treatment or over-treatment of low blood glucose reactions. This is most likely to occur in children who have had several severe hypoglycemic reactions, especially if one or more occurred in public. Extreme anxiety related to a very specific subject, such as fear of hypoglycemia among children and adolescents, can be treated quite effectively with any of several psychological treatments that come under the general heading "behavior therapy."

Common Emotional Pitfalls Among Parents

Parents, especially mothers, may be at greater risk of emotional adjustment difficulties than their sons or daughters with diabetes. In fact, it's very common that, by the time I see the family of a newly diagnosed child on the second or third day of hospitalization, the child may have already recovered from the initial emotional upheaval and trauma, whereas the parents are still tearful and very upset. The prevalence of depression among mothers of newly diagnosed youngsters increases two- to threefold in the first year after diagnosis. It may be less common, and somewhat shorter in duration, among fathers. As with adolescents, depression among parents shows itself as a cluster of symptoms that may include:

▲ Persistent sadness, perhaps accompanied by crying spells
▲ Disruption of normal sleep and appetite patterns
▲ Recurring negative thoughts about oneself
▲ Thoughts of suicide, self-harm, or running away
▲ Psychosomatic problems such as headaches or back pain

▲ Decreased mental sharpness; problems with concentration and memory

▲ Withdrawal from previously enjoyed activities or social relationships

▲ Reduced performance of household, work, or other responsibilities

Most parents who become depressed soon after the diagnosis get over it within six to nine months. Those with strong family histories of depression or a prior personal history of depression may be more likely to suffer a depressive episode during this time and to have repeat episodes later on. Depressed mothers or fathers tend to be less energetic and careful in their parenting styles than other parents, so it is important that they attend to their own needs during this period, seeking treatment for depression if necessary, to make sure that the child's needs can also be met. You can treat depression very effectively with antidepressant medications, psychotherapy, or a combination of the two, so there is no need for anyone to continue to suffer from it after it is diagnosed. Ask your doctor for a referral to a mental health professional if either you or your spouse experiences the pattern of symptoms noted above for more than a few weeks, particularly if you sense that you are not participating effectively in your child's diabetes management.

Some parents, particularly parents of young or recently diagnosed children, may be prone to an overanxious reaction to diabetes and its management. Although such families may help their child achieve excellent glucose control, it often comes at the expense of intense misery and worry. Sometimes parents excessively fear hypoglycemia in their children, resulting in many of the same symptoms children suffer when they fear hypoglycemia. It's natural for you to be walking on eggs the first few months after the diagnosis, questioning your ability to make the right decisions and take the right actions when diabetes problems come up. You may make frequent telephone calls to health care providers or use the emergency room too often. If this tension doesn't subside within a few months after the diagnosis or if you find yourself consumed by thinking and worrying about diabetes, rather than learning to relax a little bit, you should seek out a diabetes support group. Getting emotional support and suggestions from "veteran" parents and learning that you're not the only one going through this can be very helpful. If that doesn't give you some relief, it might be time to seek individual professional help.

Behavioral and psychological research on diabetes has not studied fathers to a great extent. Some studies have shown that having fathers more involved in diabetes management improves *treatment adherence* (how well the person with diabetes is able to follow the treatment plan) and diabetic control. As noted above, fathers don't seem to be as prone to depression as mothers, perhaps because many fathers often assume less of the practical and emotional burden of daily diabetes responsibilities.

In fact, studies have shown that mothers of adolescents with diabetes often experience a diabetes "burnout" syndrome, in which they withdraw from responsibility for daily diabetes management. Relinquishing some responsibility to a teenager can be a good thing if it is done carefully, systematically, and with proper consideration of the adolescent's diabetes knowledge and psychological maturity. However, if it occurs for the wrong reasons, such as the parents' anger, resentment, frustration, or fatigue, it can be a prescription for disaster. Diabetes burnout can be minimized or prevented by sharing diabetes responsibilities between the parents, honest communication when one partner is wearing out, and giving one another periodic "vacations" from diabetes duties. Be clear about which parent is on duty. Single parents may have to look to their former spouses and the child's grandparents for this type of support. Another source for a needed break, both for parents and the child, is to arrange for the child to attend a diabetes summer camp. Diabetes summer camps are available in most regions of the country, and many camps provide financial assistance for children who lack the ability to pay (see the Resources section for information on books about diabetes camp).

Parents, especially those who live far away from their children's grandparents and other relatives, are also often reluctant to leave their child in the care of others. I've seen couples who haven't been out by themselves, without their children, for several years after their child was diagnosed with diabetes. This is a bad idea for both the parents and the child. Parents deserve and need breaks from their child's diabetes. Parents should devote a minimum of a few hours per month solely to enjoying and improving their marital relationship. Everyone in the family wins when parents make the commitment to do this regularly. After all, your child needs you to have a healthy marriage so that you can be at your best as parents.

Spending some time away from your child is also a good way for you to express confidence that your youngster can begin to handle some of life's challenges without you. When you resist separating from your child, you send the message that diabetes is even more threatening and dangerous than it really is and that it presents immediate dangers to your child that you yourself must head off. For your child to grow up without an incapacitating fear of diabetes, you must express confidence that he or she can begin to handle it without you. Many families have trouble finding a sitter they can trust with this responsibility. I suggest that you use your local diabetes resources to find a teenager or adult with diabetes, or perhaps a sibling of someone with diabetes, who can care for your child on a reasonably regular basis. Another way for you to express confidence in your child, while ensuring his or her health safety, is to arrange sleepovers at the homes of other children with diabetes. I know parents who have prepared detailed "operating manuals" for their children with diabetes that include all the necessary emergency phone numbers, instructions on insulin and blood glucose tests, sample meal plans, and so forth.

Common Emotional Pitfalls Among Siblings

Because diabetes invades just about every aspect of family life, it obviously might have some effects on brothers and sisters. Siblings can play an important role in providing social support to help your child handle the challenges of living with diabetes, so it's important to try to head off any problems that might stand in the way of this. The most common negative reaction among brothers and sisters is jealousy and resentment, which could be caused by any of the following:

▲ The perception, whether real or imagined, that the child with diabetes gets more attention, is disciplined less harshly, or has more privileges

▲ Impositions on the child who doesn't have diabetes, such as changes in the family's eating habits, scheduling conflicts, and financial constraints

▲ The fear of developing diabetes themselves

▲ Feeling responsible for the onset of their sibling's diabetes

If I had the cure for sibling rivalry, I could retire a rich man. I'm not sure that it's really any worse among families of youngsters with diabetes, but diabetes often seems to serve as the stage on which it's played out. But I've also seen plenty of families in which the siblings helped, supported, and encouraged the child with diabetes. Here are some suggestions to help you promote a healthy relationship between your child with diabetes and your other children:

▲ Don't miss a chance to emphasize that diabetes is a family challenge and that all members of the family are expected to do their part to stay on top of it.

▲ Simply recognizing the risks of negative effects of diabetes on your child's brothers and sisters is an important first step.

▲ Explicitly thank your child's brothers and sisters frequently for their help and support. Periodically do something special with them or for them to show your appreciation for their cooperation and patience.

▲ Try to include all family members in the management of diabetes by giving each sibling (especially older siblings) a role to play, such as helping to keep track of supplies or helping to plan healthy meals.

▲ If you reward your child for good self-care habits, remember to reward your other children for their healthy habits, as well as for their help and support.

▲ Carefully point out to your other children that their needs or interests may also create an imposition or inconvenience for their sibling with diabetes (and not just always the other way around). It's important to do this in a sensitive and caring way, and to avoid coming across as critical and sarcastic.

For Fathers Only

Let's face it—men just aren't as emotional as women. I'm not going to get into whether this is a good or bad thing, but it clearly sets couples up for some trouble if their reactions to a serious stressful situation, such as childhood diabetes, are extremely different. The best advice I can give men is to try as hard as you can to do these things regularly:

▲ Ask your spouse how she is doing emotionally with your child's diabetes and make sure you listen.

▲ Now and then, tell your spouse how much you appreciate her efforts and point out how she is doing a good job.

▲ Periodically offer to take on more diabetes responsibility than usual.

▲ If at all possible, come to your child's diabetes clinic visits.

▲ Be actively involved in encouraging your child's cooperation with diabetes management.

I should add that the *quality* of your involvement in managing your child's diabetes may be more important than the *quantity*. Saying and doing the things I've listed above will be most helpful to your spouse when they are offered at the right times and in the right situations. Pay attention to those times when she seems most distressed or worn-out, because that is when your involvement will be the most helpful and appreciated.

Promoting Emotional Healing

I've given a sampling of the many and varied emotional reactions that diabetes can produce within families. Because these emotional challenges may seem insurmountable, some families feel awkward and tend to shrink from tackling them head on. This is precisely the wrong reaction! There are many effective methods for promoting emotional healing, such as:

▲ taking advantage of the support available from relatives, friends, or neighbors

▲ attending diabetes support groups or summer camps

▲ relying on spiritual supports

▲ gathering more information about diabetes

▲ seeking the services of a qualified mental health professional

Regardless of the specific method that works for your child and family, resolving the emotional challenges posed by diabetes is a key task that will make it much easier for you and your child to handle the tasks that follow.

Every parent knows how hard it is to watch a son or daughter go through a troubling, painful time while feeling powerless to help. You can't change the fact that your child has diabetes or free your child from the tyranny of insulin, blood glucose tests, or controlled eating, but there are some helpful things that you can do when your child hits an emotional low point.

▲ Just listen! Give your child the chance to express exactly what he or she is feeling, without interruption.

▲ Repeat back in your own words what you heard your child say.

▲ Empathize, don't analyze. Your child's feelings are valid and understandable, so don't try to argue with, dismiss, or explain them. Just acknowledge your child's pain, and try to share it if you can.

▲ Ask what you can do to help and take any suggestions seriously.

▲ Encourage emotional self-expression through outlets such as art, music, or writing.

Many youngsters and their parents find some comfort in knowing that diabetes is not an obstacle to achieving personal goals and ambitions. Here's a list of well-known, highly accomplished people with diabetes from many fields:

Ken Anderson, *NFL quarterback*

Menachem Begin, *Prime Minister of Israel*

Jack Benny, *entertainer*

Fran Carpentier, *Parade magazine editor*

Sylvia Chase, *TV Journalist*

Bobby Clarke, *NHL player and coach*

Mark Collie, *country rock musician*

Chris Dudley, *NBA center*

Thomas Edison, *inventor*

Curt Frazer, *NHL player*

Mikhail Gorbachev, *former President of the USSR*

Bill Gullickson, *major league pitcher*

Tom Hallion, *major league umpire*

Jonathan Hayes, *NFL tight end*

Howard Hughes, *industrialist*

Zippora Karz, *soloist with the New York City Ballet*

Michelle McGann, *professional golfer*

Bret Michaels, *rock singer*

Mary Tyler Moore, *actress*

Emmy Lou Packard, *artist*

Tom Parks, *comedian*

Buddy Roemer, *Governor of Louisiana*

Jean Smart, *actress*

Wade Wilson, *NFL quarterback*

Scott Verplank, *professional golfer*

TAKE-HOME MESSAGE

2 Diabetes forces your family to cope with recurring psychological and emotional challenges. If you can handle these challenges effectively, then daily life with diabetes will be more satisfying for you and your child.

KEY
3

FAMILY COMMUNICATION

Emotional Coping

Diabetes Knowledge

Erica was a 14-year-old girl whose diabetic control had been getting steadily worse for the past couple of years. Almost every day, she had serious arguments with her parents about her diabetes responsibilities. So, Erica's doctor referred the family to a psychologist. At their first session with the psychologist, Erica and her parents agreed that they wanted to be able to talk to each other more effectively about touchy issues like diabetes. They reported that they often said things like these to each other:

ERICA:
"You two never let me have own opinions about anything."

"You're always cutting down my friends!"

"Give me a break! That's a stupid thing to say!"

"You never show any trust in me at all!"

"You're always ordering me around!"

MOTHER:
"Why can't you be responsible instead of being so lazy?"

"Of course I don't trust you. You're always lying to me."

"Not one of your friends cares at all about your health."

FATHER:
'You're just trying to get back at us and to hurt us by being irresponsible."

'If you keep behaving this way you might as well kiss your vision good-bye."

Erica and her family were seen regularly by a psychologist for several months. They worked on developing better communication habits and using these to overcome their disagreements about diabetes. They reported that learning to solve problems together and to communicate in positive and constructive ways had been very helpful to them and that Erica was now far more responsible for her diabetes than in the past.

3

FAMILY
COMMUNICATION

Many researchers have asked why some families manage childhood diabetes well, while others struggle with it. The results of their studies point to the importance of family skills in *communication*, *negotiation*, and *conflict resolution*. Families who are skilled at these tasks do better with most of life's challenges, including the special ones that come with diabetes. Management of diabetes can serve as the playing field for all kinds of conflicts calling for negotiation and effective communication between children and parents. But many families have developed ineffective and counterproductive communication patterns that prevent them from solving diabetes problems effectively as a group. Dealing successfully with the challenges that come with having diabetes in the family will be easier for each of you if you are able to talk openly and honestly instead of concealing true feelings or acting them out in indirect, non-communicative ways. Open, honest, direct, and respectful family communication brings all kinds of rewards to family life. Families who communicate effectively are closer, their daily lives are more pleasant and organized, their reactions are more predictable, and they are more efficient at solving problems and tackling those big and little stresses that complicate life.

Keeping childhood diabetes in control depends heavily on three factors:

1. Your family's ability to fit the diabetes treatment tasks into your daily routines

2. How clearly the diabetes responsibilities of each family member are defined

3. How well the family members solve diabetes problems together

I suspect that high-quality family communication, both in general and about diabetes in particular, is the most important skill that successful families possess to help them accomplish these three things. Another important feature of successful families is what some family therapists call *reciprocity of positive reinforcement*. Basically, this means that there are a lot of exchanges of praise, acknowledgment, and gratitude between family members, and that these kinds of interactions outweigh those that are critical, defensive, or punishing in nature. Families who keep this positive interaction as a priority for all family relationships, not just parent-child interactions, enjoy a more satisfying and fulfilling family life. In too many families, communication about diabetes is almost entirely negative and critical, resulting all too often in avoidance of diabetes-related problems, rather than cooperation to solve those problems.

Communication, like any other skill, can be evaluated and improved. Diabetes can tax any family's communication skills because it's really hard to talk about it, yet the disease itself requires that you and your family do just that, day in and day out. Many of the families who have come to me for help over the years really seemed to have a hard time communicating their concern and caring for one another in ways that are constructive, supportive, and helpful, rather than critical and demeaning. Let's face it, youngsters often struggle with the demands and hassles that diabetes forces on them. Their parents, in turn, are often frustrated with being unable to help their sons or daughters come to terms with all of this. When it comes to talking with teenagers about really serious matters, something seems to cause many of us to forget everything we know about communicating in an open, calm, and respectful way. Just when we need our very best communication skills, those skills seem to abandon us. So being able to connect effectively with one another about these really painful and sensitive issues isn't easy, and it requires a lot of time, energy, effort, and practice to achieve.

That's what this chapter was designed to help you with. Over the past decade, I've been studying the effects of family communication training on relationships between parents and adolescents with diabetes and on the teenager's *treatment adherence* (how well he or she is able to follow the diabetes treatment plan), adjustment to diabetes, and glucose control. I'll explain what we've learned from this research, as well as what other behavioral scientists have learned about parent-adolescent communication in general. Although much of this chapter focuses on teenagers, I think this information is just as relevant for parents of younger children with diabetes. The foundations for effective family communication are formed well before your children reach adolescence, and perhaps knowing this information will help you prevent or minimize some of the common problems that often surface during adolescence. Those of you who have younger children with diabetes can benefit from this chapter by better preparing for your child's adolescence. Getting a head start on establishing good communication habits will really pay off for you later. Just as it is important for you to communicate effectively with your child who has diabetes, effective communication between parents is also crucial to successful family management of diabetes. And, if your family is among the many families who have experienced divorce, separation, or otherwise live in an "alternative" family structure, solid communication between and among the important adults in your child's life are even more essential. So, regardless of your child's age or family situation, your family can do your best with diabetes if you place a top priority on developing and maintaining healthy communication patterns, both about diabetes and about life in general.

Teaching Families to Communicate

At this point I will describe our family communication training research for you, because much of the rest of the chapter is based on what we've learned from that project, in terms of both our data and our clinical experiences with the families who took part in the project. There had been a lot of research showing that family conflict, especially parent-adolescent conflict, was associated consistently with poor treatment adherence and poor diabetic control. Other studies showed that effective family communication and negotiation skills and strong family cohesiveness were important factors in achieving good diabetes control. My colleagues and I reasoned that we could help families get on top of their child's diabetes more effectively by helping them improve their communication and conflict resolution skills.

In our first major study, we recruited 119 families of adolescents with diabetes in St. Louis, Missouri and Jacksonville, Florida who told us that their teen-parent relationships had more than an average amount of friction about both general issues and diabetes. Each family was then assigned by chance either to continue with their regular medical care or to receive either of two extra treatments. About a third of the families participated in ten sessions of a multi-family support group. During every group session, they received advanced diabetes education about a particular diabetes-related issue and then they discussed their problems and successes in dealing with that issue. Another third of the families participated in ten sessions of family communication training using an approach called *behavioral family systems therapy* (BFST). This method had been used effectively with distressed families of delinquent teenagers, teenaged girls with eating disorders, and hyperactive adolescents, so we decided to test it with families who were struggling with diabetes. In BFST, the psychologist acts like a teacher or coach. While observing the family's discussion of a conflict-ridden issue, the psychologist interrupts to give feedback to family members about their communication errors and positive communication habits, instructs them in more constructive ways of communicating, and has them rehearse the new skills in sessions. The families are also given behavioral homework assignments to do between sessions so they could practice their new skills and enhance their chances for making lasting changes. Every family in our study completed questionnaires about teen-parent conflict and communication patterns.

They were interviewed now and then by telephone about disputes or arguments that had occurred the day before, and they were tape-recorded during family sessions while discussing issues that had been the source of recent friction within the family. We learned a lot from being able to observe and listen to these families so closely. Our results showed that, compared with the support group or with regular medical care alone, BFST produced more improvements in teen-parent relationships and family communication. When we looked at outcomes that were specific to diabetes, such as the adolescents' treatment adherence and their glucose control, we found that general improvements in teen-parent relationships translated into better diabetes outcomes for the younger girls (12 to 14 years old) and for boys of any age (12 to 17 years old) in our sample. The older girls (14 to 17 years old) didn't seem to benefit as much in terms of improved treatment adherence or diabetic control. We also found that one year after treatment, those who received the BFST treatment continued to have better teen-parent relationships and better diabetes treatment adherence than those in the other two groups. We are now in the midst of a second major study in which we have made some changes to BFST that are designed to increase its impact on treatment adherence and glucose control. We are optimistic that this research will result in a systematic and well-defined intervention that can be helpful to many families in the future. In the meantime, this chapter gives you many of the basic steps of the BFST treatment so that you can improve your family's communication skills.

With the BFST, we have shown that it is possible to evaluate and improve the communication skills of families of teenagers with diabetes and that, in many cases, doing this helps families cope more effectively with diabetes. This information may help you size up and improve your family's communication skills or determine whether this is an area that your family needs some help with. By taking a close look at your family's communication patterns and working together toward a goal of improvement in your problem areas, each of you can develop stronger skills in resolving conflicts and negotiating solutions to disagreements.

Sizing Up Family Communication

Families have personalities, just like people do, and they tend to develop persistent characteristics that color many of their functions and interactions. Our research, as well as that of others, points to three aspects of the family that each play a key role in determining how well the family is able to communicate about day-to-day problems, negotiate acceptable solutions to disagreements or conflicts, and maintain healthy and positive relationships during the trying adolescent period. They are:

1. The effectiveness of family communication skills

2. The extent to which family members hold extreme or irrational attitudes or beliefs about each others' behavior and motives

3. The degree to which the family's rules, boundaries, and decision making are structured in ways that preserve parental unity and authority while allowing gradually increasing independence by the adolescent

Let's take a closer look at each of these family characteristics to help you evaluate your family's "personality" and to begin to identify areas that may need some extra attention and effort.

Communication Skills

Every family has disagreements. When the same disagreements or disputes happen over and over again, they tend to get blown out of proportion. When you seem to be covering the same ground again and again, it may be a sign that your family, as a group, needs to learn how to approach the conflict with the idea of resolving it. Are there situations in your family that seem to keep popping up as causes of arguments and friction? If so, here's a list of rules for fair fighting that you might be able to use in these situations, whether the issue relates to diabetes or not. These basic rules are a good starting point for most families to begin work on improving their ability to solve problems together.

▲ *Schedule your fights.* Instead of tangling with one another when you're most upset, pick a time and place that you all agree on and devote about an hour exclusively to talking through and resolving your disagreement. Most people solve problems together much more effectively if they're not already very upset. Putting some time and space between when the problem happened and your discussion about it gives you a chance to think through your points, mull over the position of the others involved, and perhaps come up with compromise solutions that you can suggest. Some families have better success having their discussions in a restaurant, a park, or some other public place.

▲ *Stay on the topic.* Conversations that stray from the main topic tend to be unproductive, confusing, and distracting rather than leading the group to a consensus. Start these conversations with a statement such as, "Let's talk about how we're always having arguments about your blood sugar results," and then stick to the topic that you have chosen.

▲ *Use "I" statements.* Avoid beginning your comments with blaming and accusing "you" statements, such as "You've screwed up again," and "You never listen to what I have to say." These kinds of statements often put the other person on the defensive and thus obstruct further communication. Instead, using "I" statements helps you retain control of our own thoughts and feelings, and you avoid blaming the other person for your reactions. Examples of "I" statements are "I'm upset that this still isn't getting done right even though we've talked it over several times," and "I get worried about your health when I find out that you didn't take your insulin when it was scheduled."

▲ *Be honest and fair.* Avoid using absolute terms such as "always" and "never." When estimating the frequencies of errors and failures, do so as accurately as possible. These absolutes are usually not true, and using them often has one of two bad effects: the other person gets busy thinking up exceptions to the statement or using these words to inflame the situation even more. Both of these results get in the way of healthy communication and effective problem solving.

▲ *Make sure that you understand each other.* Make a habit of saying things like "Now tell me what you believe we've agreed to do from now on," or "Let me make sure that I understand you. Did you say that _____?"

▲ *Keep the discussion in the present and the future.* Avoid dwelling on another's failures or mistakes that occurred in the past. Refer to past problems only to the extent that you're providing information that can be used constructively in the future. Remember that change can only occur in the future and that you can't change what has happened in the past. So try to keep your discussion in the present and future.

▲ *Avoid interrupting.* Respect the speaker's right to finish his or her statements without interruption. If necessary, use an object to symbolize who has the floor, and don't speak until the object has been passed to you.

Errors

Researchers have identified some common communication errors among parents and adolescents, errors that I often see in the families I'm working with clinically. Once your family is able to conduct a successful "fair fight" according to the rules I laid out above, then it may be time for you to move on to addressing some of your family's communication errors. These can really interfere with getting your point heard. There are often much more productive ways to make your point than the ways you find most comfortable and familiar. You will recognize that some of the statements below are obviously made mostly by parents and others mostly by adolescents. It's a good idea to begin by recognizing that communication problems lie in interactions between people, not in problems that are within people.

ERROR: Yelling, name calling, swearing

Example: "You're a stupid jerk if that's what you think!"
Why it's a problem: It tends to cause anger, it is unproductive, and it cuts off further communication.
Alternative: "I have a hard time understanding your point of view on this."

ERROR: Interrupting

Example: Interjecting one's own statements and objections before waiting for the other person to finish speaking.

Why it's a problem: It tends to create an angry reaction and cuts off further communication. It communicates a lack of interest in understanding the other person's point.

Alternative: Come up with a simple gesture or signal that family members can use to indicate when they are finished speaking

ERROR: Communicating through another person

Example: "Mom, tell Dad that I don't want him coming to my doctor's appointments anymore."

Why it's a problem: It shows a lack of trust or confidence in the person for whom the communication is really intended, and it runs the risk that the intent of the communication will be lost in the translation.

Alternative: Speak directly to the person with whom you are communicating, or ask for help in doing so through a statement such as "Mom, can you help me tell Dad that I'd rather he didn't come to my doctor's appointments anymore?"

Self-Monitoring Your Errors

Now that you have some clear communication goals to strive for, you can take some practical steps to get there. Start by having each family member "self-monitor" his or her own communication errors. It isn't easy to do this because none of us want to admit that we make mistakes. To make this self-monitoring most successful, try to keep it private at first. Don't point out or count each other's errors—yet.

During a family meeting, have each family member choose, with the help of other family members, one communication error to target for improvement. Count and record the number of times you catch yourself making the communication error that you've targeted. Keep a detailed diary in which you record the who, what, when, where, and how of each occurrence of the error. This will help you recognize patterns in your behavior and what triggers your responses.

Self-monitoring often helps correct problem habits that people want to change. But if it doesn't work, there are a few more steps you and your family can take:

▲ Monitor one another's communication errors and successes using the same basic approaches given above. At first, it's best to write down the instances of errors and discuss them later during a family meeting rather than give each other immediate critical feedback.

▲ Sometimes it's better to give a name or label to the communication error(s) that you're working on. It's a little easier for people to receive feedback such as "That was interrupting" instead of "You just interrupted me again!"

▲ After your family is comfortable with giving and receiving feedback about your communication habits, you may want to set up a simple system of rewards for meeting communication goals or minor fines for communication errors.

If these kinds of steps don't work, look for help from a mental health professional, preferably one with training, experience, and credentials in family therapy.

Extreme Beliefs

Let's face it, all of us have some strong attitudes and opinions that aren't very well based in facts, and we tend to hang on to them as if they were priceless gems. People are prone to various errors in logic and often come to faulty conclusions that color their reactions to their experiences. Nowhere has this been more obvious than when I've talked with parents and adolescents about how they view one another's behavior and motives. For example, if I ask a family to discuss a disagreement they've been having repeatedly, it's going to be a lot harder for them to keep a cool head, to understand one another's points of view, and to take others' suggestions seriously if they think things like these about each other:

▲ "You don't want me to have any friends."

▲ "You're only doing this to hurt us."

- ▲ "There is no way you could ever understand me."
- ▲ "Everyone who behaves this way ends up destroying their lives."
- ▲ "You only made up this rule to get back at me."
- ▲ "All teenagers must obey their parents perfectly."

Sound familiar? We all have ideas like these some of the time, but it's important that you be able to step back and examine your attitudes, identify those that are driving your behavior, and see whether there is some way that you could soften or temper your beliefs so that communication can proceed a little more smoothly. There are some common "extreme beliefs" held by parents and adolescents, which I describe below. I provide a softened restatement of the same belief that might lower the emotional temperature of family conversations. Have you identified a trouble spot in need of an attitude adjustment?

EXTREME	BELIEF EXAMPLE	SOFTENED BELIEF
Ruination	All kids who behave like this have long-term complications of diabetes someday.	If we keep working together as a family, we'll turn things around.
Perfectionism	My youngster must do every diabetes task perfectly.	Nobody's perfect. I don't think I could do all of these things everyday.
Malicious intent	You only did this to get back at us for our rules.	Not everything kids do is done for or to their parents.
Conventionalism	We have to do things just like other families.	Our lives will be easier if we learn how to adapt diabetes to our family instead of the opposite.
Obedience	Teenagers must always obey their parents.	I wasn't perfect when I was a kid, and I turned out okay.
Unfairness	It isn't fair that I have to live with all these rules.	The world is full of rules. What right do I have to be so special?

Maybe you're still having trouble really accepting a softened version of an attitude, and you want to know what else you can do. Here are a few techniques that you can use separately or together that might be of help:

- ▲ Try *reframing*, which means viewing the situation from a different, more positive perspective. For example, instead of wondering why your daughter isn't more responsible and mature toward her diabetes care, perhaps you could focus on the fact that she has never been hospitalized and that she hasn't let diabetes stand in the way of her goals in school and sports.

- ▲ Remember your own adolescence.

- ▲ Conduct an experiment: Ask some adults with well-controlled diabetes how they behaved as teenagers.

- ▲ Simulate living with diabetes for a few days or a week to see how well you do with it. Test your blood glucose three times a day, eat on schedule according to a written meal plan, deny yourself any foods not in your meal plan, and inject yourself with sterile saline before breakfast, lunch, and supper. Afterward, remember that your child's diabetes doesn't go away after a few days.

Family Structure

Even if a family has good basic communication skills and entirely reasonable beliefs and attitudes about each other, it's possible that they might not be able to use these skills effectively to solve problems together. This can happen when the usual lines of authority and influence within the family have been undermined. Healthy family structure requires that the parents are a reasonably unified and cohesive unit and that each contributes to and supports decisions and family rules affecting the children. Healthy families maintain clear boundaries between the parents and the children, and influence within the family flows primarily from the parents to the children, with an increasing voice for the children as they grow and mature.

There are problems with family structure and functioning that commonly cause families to have trouble using their communication skills effectively. Single-parent and blended families may be at somewhat greater risk of these problems, but no family is immune. Although fewer families have this type of problem than the difficulties of poor communication skills and extreme beliefs, those who do tend to have considerable problems in coping with diabetes.

▲ *Weak parental coalitions:* In some families, the parents just aren't on the same side as far as discipline, limit setting, and parent-adolescent boundaries. For example, the father may allow the child with diabetes to eat whatever she pleases, whereas the mother may be very strict about consistently following the dietitian's recommendations. When children and adolescents sense this situation, they face the temptation of manipulating it to their advantage.

▲ *Triangulation:* This occurs when one member of the family is caught between two or more other family members who are in conflict, and each is competing for that person's support or allegiance. This problem often surfaces in families who are suffering through serious marital discord and can involve a changing cast of family members. Commonly, estranged parents compete for a child's allegiance by showering the child with gifts and privileges while prodding the child for information about the other parent's private life. It is difficult to get the kind of family cooperation that supports good diabetes management while this type of problem exists.

▲ *Cross-generational coalitions:* This is similar to triangulation, but it refers to a stable pattern in which a child and one parent consistently align themselves together as a team against the other parent. It prevents normal boundaries and lines of influence within the family and often places the parents in situations where the child can manipulate one parent against the other.

▲ *Adolescent involvement in marital discord:* This is a very common problem in families who are either experiencing marital problems or are having problems readjusting to their new lives after a divorce or separation. Unfortunately, it is also common for these youngsters to have chronically poor diabetic control. A particularly high-risk situation exists when the adolescent with diabetes threatens to go to live with the other parent whenever the custodial parent asserts limits, rules, or expectations that the teenager has trouble accepting. Youngsters who jump from one parent's home to the other can effectively blackmail their parents into giving them their way. Along with the added stress to the adolescent if the parents continue to have major post-divorce conflicts, this situation almost guarantees that the teenager will have serious problems maintaining adequate treatment adherence and glucose control.

If you believe that your family may have one or more of these problems based on family structure, it's probably interfering with your ability to deal effectively with your child's diabetes. I suggest that you seek out a psychologist or other psychotherapist who is trained and experienced in marital and family therapy to help you sort through these issues. To be resolved, these troubles usually require more than self-help fixes.

Dealing with Deception

There is a common problem in family communication that deserves its own discussion. Many youngsters with diabetes find it necessary to deceive their parents or members of their health care team in any of a variety of ways. It's hard to say how common this is, but I suspect that most youngsters with diabetes fall into this trap now and then. Deception can take many forms, including:

▲ Trading healthy school lunch foods prepared by mom for cake, cookies, candy, or doughnuts that other kids have brought

▲ Writing down bogus blood glucose results in the logbook

▲ Figuring out ways to fool the blood glucose meter, such as:

  ■ testing sibling's blood

  ■ diluting the blood with water

  ■ putting too little blood on the test strip

  ■ getting a readout before the required test time is up

  ■ reusing old strips that were in the normal range

■ using calibration strips to enter a result rather than doing a test

Modern glucose meters are less likely to allow some of these methods, but I've never ceased to be amazed at the ingenuity and creativity kids can show in figuring out ways to fool these machines.

▲ Varying the insulin dose without telling anyone about it

▲ Skipping a scheduled test because it's likely that the blood glucose is high

Deceptive behaviors like these illustrate many features of ineffective or disordered communication. First, these actions aren't honest or fair to the other members of the family or to the health care professionals who are involved, and show a lack of trust in them. Second, they are indirect and fail to send a clear message. Third, once this kind of behavior is discovered, as it inevitably is, there tends to be lots of conflict and tension about the dishonesty itself rather than resolving issues about the treatment regimen that are the core of the dispute. Why are deception and dishonesty so common among youngsters with diabetes? Is there some physical effect of diabetes that causes children to be dishonest? Does diabetes happen primarily to people who lack a conscience and solid moral values? I don't think so, because neither of these possibilities explains why the majority of youngsters with diabetes are ordinarily honest, truthful, and principled young people when it comes to everything except diabetes. I think the answers lie in other areas. Children and adolescents have a strong desire to receive approval and to avoid disapproval from their parents and from health care professionals. At the same time, a child's behavior tends to be more controlled by immediate consequences than an adult's behavior. Together, these two influences may at times cause some children to set aside their desire to be completely honest about their diabetes self-care habits to avoid disapproval and/or obtain approval from adults, even if it promises to be brief.

The treatment responsibilities expected of youngsters with diabetes may be beyond the self-control capabilities of many children and adolescents. Dishonesty may be a sign that you're expecting too much of your child in the area of diabetes responsibilities. Being truthful about lapses in self-care responsibilities often results in critical or punishing responses from adults. Even with sound treatment adherence, adolescents never have perfect control of their blood glucose. Raging hormones and psychological stress can both interfere with glucose control, even when a teenager completes other aspects of treatment carefully. This can get pretty discouraging, and many adolescents become ashamed of their self-management "failures." Abnormally high or low blood glucose is often referred to as bad, whereas those in the normal range are viewed as good. I've even observed this pattern among children who are still in the hospital a few days after diagnosis. Because treatment of diabetes consists mostly of self-management, it is understandable why children who don't achieve good diabetic control might view themselves as self-management failures who are solely to blame for their abnormal blood glucose.

Some of these problems could probably be reduced or prevented if parents and health care professionals, ideally from the moment of the diagnosis on, would learn to value honesty and partnership with these youngsters as much as they value near-normal blood glucose values. Children who come to you openly and honestly with bad news about their blood glucose or to describe a problem with staying with the meal plan are coming to you for help and guidance. It doesn't take too many exchanges that produce critical or suspicious comments from parents or health care professionals to convince most children to give up on that approach. The only "good" blood glucose value is one that is obtained accurately and acted on appropriately. When dishonesty or deception occurs, it might as well be treated as a breakdown of the diabetes care partnership among the child, parents, and health care team than as evidence of the youngster's immorality or lack of self-control. Instead, if the deception can be seen as proof of a communication problem that resides among several people, not within only one of them, it's often possible for these events to become positive growth experiences that eventually lead to a stronger diabetes partnership.

Family Meetings

I'm an advocate of regular family meetings, especially for families who are suffering with recurring problems in diabetes management.

So I encourage you to begin a habit of having regularly scheduled family meetings to review your family's rules and expectations, to discuss problem areas, and, in particular, to evaluate how things are going with your child's diabetes. Some common diabetes issues that you might consider putting on your agenda are:

▲ Your youngster's self-care behaviors, such as blood glucose testing, insulin injections, and meal plan

▲ Diabetes and school

▲ The effect of diabetes on relationships with friends and siblings

You can adjust the frequency of these meetings to your needs, but I suggest weekly for families with frequent conflict, monthly for those with minor or sporadic trouble dealing with diabetes, and perhaps every three months for those who are coasting along pretty well. I don't think too many problems get resolved when people are intensely angry with each other, so discussing disagreements or recurring problems in a calm, well-established setting is often helpful.

Here are some suggested guidelines for holding your family meetings. Set them at a time when all family members can be there, and require attendance, except for children younger than six or seven. Rotate the responsibility for running the meeting among the parents and older children. Diabetes, schoolwork, and chores should be routine agenda items, and any family member should be allowed to put other items on the agenda. Make it clear what topic is under discussion, and do your best to stay with that topic. If a new, important issue comes up, consider adding it to the agenda for later in the meeting or for a future meeting.

Family meetings are a good time to practice using the communication skills discussed earlier in this chapter. Respect the right of one person to speak at a time. If anyone becomes upset during the meeting, take a short break before returning to the discussion. The emphasis should be on calm and composed communication and problem solving. If necessary, pass around an object that symbolizes who has the floor, or have the speaker stand up. Spend no more than 15 minutes on any one agenda item, and try to end each discussion with a specific action plan. One particularly creative family came up with the idea of having their teenaged daughter keep a small tape recorder with her diabetes equipment, which she would use to audibly record her blood glucose test results and the amount of insulin she gave. Her mother agreed to write down the information from her recordings every evening.

TAKE-HOME MESSAGE

3

Effective family communication is essential for healthy adaptation to diabetes, and it becomes even more important during adolescence. You can improve your family communication skills, but you must keep this as a top family priority.

KEY
4

FAMILY SHARING OF DIABETES RESPONSIBILITIES

Family Communication

Emotional Coping

Diabetes Knowledge

Eduardo was a 10-year-old boy with diabetes who lived with his mother and his three younger sisters. His diabetic control had gotten much worse in the past few months. He and his mother were referred for additional diabetes education.

The diabetes educator learned that there had been several major changes in Eduardo's family life recently. His mother's boyfriend had moved out and his mother had taken on a second job to make ends meet. Eduardo was also much more responsible for his diabetes self-care and he was now in charge of drawing up and giving his own insulin injections. The diabetes educator suspected that Eduardo had too much responsibility and that he couldn't handle it all.

The diabetes educator helped Eduardo's mother find ways to build more adult supervision into his daily life, especially regarding his diabetes treatment. His grandmother began checking on him and helping him figure out his insulin doses. A school nurse made sure that he checked his blood sugar and took an insulin injection before he ate breakfast at school. Eduardo's diabetic control has improved greatly since these changes were made.

FAMILY SHARING OF DIABETES RESPONSIBILITIES

In working your way through the first three chapters, you have put some of the fundamentals behind you. You understand the importance of a solid foundation of diabetes knowledge and coping with the emotional side of diabetes. You've learned about the importance of firm family communication and have been introduced to some ways of improving your family's ability to negotiate and resolve conflicts. Now it's time to move on to some key tasks that are more specialized and unique to diabetes. The first of these keys is to make sure that your family achieves a healthy balance between parent responsibilities and child responsibilities regarding diabetes care. Having this balance will ensure your child's safety while helping your child make steady progress toward increasing diabetes skills, self-confidence, and autonomy.

The basic role of all parents is to help their children become independent, healthy adults. Your child's diabetes complicates, and maybe magnifies, this basic obligation, but it doesn't change it. When it comes to diabetes self-management, parents and the other members of the child's health care team are faced with some difficult decisions about how and when to shift responsibility for self-care tasks from the parent to the child. Giving your son or daughter too little responsibility could make the child feel inadequate and create self-doubts and anxiety about his or her ability to assume responsibility later. Giving your child too much responsibility too soon can lead to dangerous treatment errors and the experience of failure in early self-management efforts. This could be discouraging and may cause both you and your child to feel that it is useless to really try to keep diabetes in good control. Do you think your child has the right amount of responsibility for diabetes self-care? If not, how can you and your child get to that point? These are the kind of issues that I will try to clear up for you in this chapter.

The transfer of diabetes responsibility from parents to children is a complicated process that we are only beginning to understand. In this chapter, I present the results of several research studies that relate to the parent-child division of diabetes responsibilities. I also give some practical guidance about how much responsibility is typical for children at different ages and some suggestions about how to shift the responsibility for diabetes tasks from parent to child as safely and productively as possible. These topics are near and dear to my heart and have been the subject of several of my research studies in the past few years.

Acquiring Skills and the Steps Toward Independence

First, let's discuss how children learn diabetes skills. One study involved surveying 648 parents of children and adolescents with diabetes between the ages of 3 and 18 years about their children's performance in a wide variety of specific diabetes skills. Parents at seven pediatric medical centers were asked to indicate whether their children had mastered each skill, which we defined as the ability to complete the task correctly without any help or prompting from others. Pages 67–68 show the questionnaire that parents completed, called the Diabetes Independence Survey. When this survey was first developed in the mid-1990s, very few children or adolescents were using insulin pumps and so the survey items did not include any of the skills involved in pump use. If your child uses an insulin pump, some of the items related to insulin use may not apply directly to your daily diabetes management. The same can probably be said of modern approaches to diet in the diabetes regimen, especially the use of carbohydrate counting. Nonetheless, I think that the results of this study can still give some useful guidance about the typical ages at which kids with diabetes master the skills involved in their treatment and the order in which the skills are learned.

If your child has had diabetes for at least six months (I don't recommend using it for children who have had diabetes for less than six months), you can use this questionnaire to estimate your child's progress and then compare it to the large sample of children that we studied at the seven diabetes clinics. To answer, read each item and decide whether your child has mastered that skill. Remember that the questionnaire is designed to measure what your child is capable of, not necessarily what your child does every day, so disregard your child's cooperation with treatment when you answer. For example, your daughter may be perfectly capable of doing a blood glucose test with a meter very carefully and precisely, but she may only be doing about half as many tests as her doctor would like. In that case, you would answer yes to the item "Completes a blood glucose test using a meter." Be as truthful as possible, and if you're not sure about a certain skill, you should see if your child can actually do it before you answer. After you've answered each item, then look at the second table to help you to evaluate your child's diabetes skill mastery.

Diabetes Independence Survey: Parent Form

Instructions: For each of the following diabetes skills, please check YES if your child has mastered that skill or NO if your child has not mastered that skill. Mastery of a given skill means that your child can perform it correctly without any kind of help from another person. Please remember that we are interested in what your child can do and not in what he or she actually does. Try to ignore your child's cooperation with treatment as you fill out this survey.

DOES/CAN YOUR CHILD	YES	NO
1. Recognize symptoms of low blood glucose and tell someone about it?	☐	☐
2. Treat low blood glucose by eating something with sugar in it?	☐	☐
3. Know when a low blood glucose reaction might happen and do something to keep it from happening?	☐	☐

DOES/CAN YOUR CHILD	YES	NO
4. Know that symptoms of high blood glucose may include extreme thirst, more urination than normal, nausea, vomiting, and fatigue?	☐	☐
5. Know some actions to take to lower high blood glucose?	☐	☐
6. Know when blood glucose may be going too high and do something to keep it from happening?	☐	☐
7. Know why it is important to wear some kind of diabetes identification?	☐	☐
8. Complete a urine ketone test?	☐	☐
9. Prick a finger with a lancet to get a drop of blood for blood glucose tests?	☐	☐
10. Complete a blood glucose test using a meter?	☐	☐
11. Write down test results in a logbook?	☐	☐
12. State each type of insulin he/she uses?	☐	☐
13. State each insulin dose he/she uses?	☐	☐
14. State the times at which insulin is to be taken each day?	☐	☐
15. Draw up an injection of only one type of insulin?	☐	☐
16. Draw up an injection using a mixture of two types of insulin?	☐	☐
17. Give himself/herself an insulin injection?	☐	☐
18. Use a different site for each insulin injection?	☐	☐
19. Write down insulin types and doses in a logbook?	☐	☐
20. State the peak action of each type of insulin that he/she uses?	☐	☐
21. For each type of insulin used, state how long that insulin works?	☐	☐
22. Adjust insulin doses according to how high or low the blood glucose is?	☐	☐
23. State reasons for a need to change his/her insulin dose?	☐	☐
24. Categorize food into food groups?	☐	☐
25. Use a meal plan?	☐	☐
26. Use a meal plan in restaurants or cafeterias?	☐	☐
27. Adjust how much he/she eats according to how high or low blood glucose is?	☐	☐
28. State reasons for changing the prescribed diet?	☐	☐
29. State the role of diet in treating diabetes?	☐	☐
30. State that activities like running, swimming, cycling, and racket sports are the best kinds of exercise for people with diabetes?	☐	☐
31. Plan daily exercise according to how and when meals and injections are taken?	☐	☐
32. Adjust amount of exercise if blood glucose is unusually high or low?	☐	☐
33. Know that exercise should be avoided if he/she is sick or has ketones in his/her urine?	☐	☐
34. State two safety precautions about exercise for people with diabetes?	☐	☐
35. State some foods that are good to eat before exercising?	☐	☐

Looking at the results of the Diabetes Independence Survey (see Table 4-1. Results of the Diabetes Independence Survey, Parent Form) can give you a reasonable estimate of whether your child is gaining diabetes knowledge and skills at rates that are similar to other children in the same age range. Let's look at your child's mastery of individual skills in comparison to the children who were in our study. Table 4-1 below shows the age ranges at which 25%, 50%, and 75% of parents reported that their children had mastered each of the diabetes skills. By reading the numbers next to each item, you can understand the age ranges at which the skills are likely to be mastered. For example, for skill 5, "Know(s) some actions to take to lower high blood glucose," 25% of parents of 4-year-olds, 50% of parents of 7-year-olds, and 75% of parents of 8-year-olds reported that their children had mastered that skill. For skill 18, "Give(s) himself/herself an insulin injection," 25% of parents of 5-year-olds, 50% of parents of 8-year-olds, and 75% of parents of 10-year-olds reported that their children had mastered that skill. You should note any skills for which your child appears to have much later or much earlier mastery than other children in the same age-group and discuss these with your doctor and diabetes educator.

Table 4-1. **Results of the Diabetes Independence Survey, Parent Form**
For each item, the table presents the age at which 25%, 50%, and 75% of parents of youths with type 1 diabetes reported that their children had mastered that skill.

DOES/CAN YOUR CHILD	25%	50%	75%
1. Recognize symptoms of low blood glucose and tell someone about it?	3 years old	4 years old	5 years old
2. Treat low blood glucose by eating something with sugar in it?	3	4	7
3. Know when a low blood glucose reaction might happen and do something to keep it from happening?	6	7	10
4. Know that symptoms of high blood glucose may include extreme thirst, more urination than normal, nausea, vomiting, and fatigue?	6	7	9
5. Know some actions to take to lower high blood glucose?	4	7	8
6. Know when blood glucose may be going too high and do something to keep it from happening?	7	10	15

Table 4-1. continued

DOES/CAN YOUR CHILD	25%	50%	75%
7. Know why it is important to wear some kind of diabetes identification?	3	4	7
8. Complete a urine ketone test?	6	8	14
9. Prick a finger with a lancet to get a drop of blood for blood glucose tests?	4	5	6
10. Complete a blood glucose test using a meter?	4	6	7
11. Write down test results in a logbook?	6	7	9
12. State each type of insulin he/she uses?	6	8	9
13. State each insulin dose he/she uses?	7	10	10
14. State the times at which insulin is to be taken each day?	4	5	6
15. Draw up an injection of only one type of insulin?	7	8	10
16. Draw up an injection using a mixture of two types of insulin?	7	10	11
17. Give himself/herself an insulin injection?	5	8	10
18. Use a different site for each insulin injection?	3	6	8
19. Write down insulin type and dose in a logbook?	7	8	11
20. State the peak of action of each type of insulin that he/she uses?	10	13	18+
21. For each type of insulin used, state how long that insulin works?	10	14	18+
22. Adjust insulin doses according to how high or low the blood glucose is?	10	13	18+
23. State reasons for a need to change his/her insulin dose?	7	8	12
24. Categorize food into food groups?	4	6	8
25. Use a meal plan?	7	9	14
26. Use a meal plan in restaurants or cafeterias?	7	10	18+
27. Adjust how much he/she eats according to how high or low the blood glucose is?	7	9	14
28. State reasons for changing the prescribed diet?	7	10	14
29. State the role of diet in treating diabetes?	5	7	11
30. State that activities like running, swimming, cycling, and racket sports are the best kinds of exercise for people with diabetes?	6	7	9
31. Plan daily exercise according to how and when meals and injections are taken?	10	12	18+
32. Adjust amount of exercise if blood glucose is unusually high or low?	7	9	11
33. Know that exercise should be avoided if he/she is sick or has ketones in his/her urine?	6	10	15
34. State two safety precautions about exercise for people with diabetes?	8	10	16
35. State some foods that are good to eat before exercising?	6	10	10

One thing you should take away from this survey is that, for any given diabetes skill, children master that skill at widely varying ages. For example, parents in our study reported that doing a blood glucose test with a meter was mastered by 25% of 5 year-olds, 50% of 8 year-olds, and 75% of 10 year-olds. For more complex skills, there could be an even wider age range. For example, parents reported that knowing that exercise should be avoided if there are ketones in the urine was mastered by 25% of 8 year-olds, 50% of 10 year-olds, and 75% of 15 year-olds. This means that, for many diabetes skills, we can't simply say that "All 10 year-olds should give their own insulin injections," or "All 14 year-olds should be able to adjust their own insulin doses based on their blood glucose levels." You have to leave room for individual differences among children, taking into account such things as your child's learning ability, attention and concentration, judgment, emotional responsibility, and other such characteristics when deciding how much responsibility your child should have.

Comparing children to others of the same age is one way to judge whether a child is progressing normally, but we all know that children of a certain age can vary tremendously in learning ability, social judgment, and emotional maturity. Now comes a harder question: Is your child's level of self-care responsibility appropriate to your child's level of *psychological* maturity? Unfortunately, I can't give a simple, clear-cut answer to this question. Instead, I'm going to tell you about another study we conducted to explore this issue. To make things simple, I'll give you the main findings first, so that you don't get too lost in all of the scientific details I summarize for you below. We found that children who had more diabetes responsibility than other children at the same level of psychological maturity had far worse diabetes outcomes. The children with too much self-care responsibility were less likely than other children to complete their treatment responsibilities consistently, were in worse diabetic control, and were more likely to be hospitalized due to diabetes. Now let me back up and help you understand how we did this study.

We wanted to explore what happens to diabetic control and treatment adherence (how well the person with diabetes is able to follow the treatment plan) when children have just enough, too much, or too little responsibility for diabetes treatment and monitoring tasks. We evaluated 100 children with diabetes between the ages of 5 and 17 with tests of psychological maturity and tests of diabetes self-care responsibility. Then we calculated the ratio of each child's level of diabetes self-care responsibility to his or her psychological maturity level. This resulted in a measure of how appropriate the child's diabetes responsibility was to his or her level of psychological maturity. We divided the children into three groups based on this score: those with too much, too little, or just enough diabetes responsibility compared with their psychological maturity.

We then asked whether the children in these three groups differed in terms of treatment adherence, knowledge of diabetes, diabetic control, and hospitalizations. Our results showed that children with too much self-care responsibility had all kinds of problems: worse diabetes knowledge, poorer treatment adherence, more hospitalizations, and poorer diabetic control. The children with too little and just enough self-care autonomy were much less likely to have these problems. We found no evidence that children with less responsibility than they were capable of were any different in terms of diabetes outcomes than those who had just the right amount of responsibility.

These findings challenged the traditional view that more diabetes independence is always better and suggested that we should be careful not to encourage too much diabetes independence too soon among children and adolescents. It's not easy for parents to match their children's self-care responsibility to their maturity perfectly, so it's probably best to err on the side of too much parental responsibility rather than too little. Overall, we concluded that families in which the parents have managed to stay involved in diabetes management during adolescence may achieve better diabetes outcomes. And guess what? I'm reasonably sure that the families who manage to do this are the same ones who have fairly solid communication skills like those discussed in the previous chapter. Later on, I share a few ideas about how parents can stay involved in their adolescent's diabetes management in ways that are helpful and supportive, and less likely to create friction and conflict.

Like a lot of research studies, this one raised as many questions as it answered. For one, we didn't follow children over a long period; we simply took a snapshot of where they were at one point in time. It's possible that we would reach different conclusions if we studied a group of children for several years. For example, maybe making a few mistakes on the road to diabetes independence isn't always a bad thing. For many children, coming into contact with the logical, natural consequences of lapses in responsibility might be a valuable learning experience. But for now, our findings suggest that parents and health care professionals should be careful not to expect children and adolescents with diabetes to take on too much responsibility too soon. When youngsters are in poor diabetic control or aspects of diabetes self-care aren't getting done according to plan, it might be wise to ask yourself whether you're expecting too much of your child.

Transferring Diabetes Responsibilities to Your Child

Giving too much diabetes care responsibility too soon may be risky, so how do you go about transferring responsibility to your child in safe and productive ways? How can you stay involved in your teenager's diabetes management in ways that are helpful and constructive, rather than intrusive and insulting? There are some practical guidelines you may find useful.

Because it's always helpful to know what you're aiming for, I outline what I believe is the most successful approach to encouraging safe self-care independence among children and adolescents with diabetes. There are three basic characteristics of families that determine whether this process is smooth, comfortable, and satisfying, or is frustrating, conflict ridden, and ineffective. These characteristics are:

1. How the parents and health care team react to the child's mistakes and failures in diabetes self-care
2. The effectiveness of communication among the child, the parents, and the health care team about self-care responsibilities
3. The degree to which parents are effective skill trainers

Actions and Reactions

One of the most important factors that affects the transfer of diabetes self-care responsibilities is how parents and the diabetes health care team respond to the child's inevitable mistakes, errors in judgment, and lapses in responsibility. When the child must face excessively critical, punitive, or belittling responses by adults, especially regarding failures that are at the limits of the child's capabilities, this often conveys to the child a sense of futility and helplessness. Parents who can find something positive to say about their child's efforts, who can view the child's failure as partially the parent's responsibility, and who can view errors as a painful but natural part of the learning process are more likely to find that their children accept diabetes self-management responsibilities more smoothly.

Proper Communications

A successful transfer of responsibility for any diabetes skill from parent to child requires a partnership consisting of the parent, the child, and the diabetes health care team. So, the second key ingredient is regular and effective communication among all three parties regarding the who, what, why, how, and when of each aspect of diabetes self-management. Ideally, this would include:

- ▲ Goal setting *with*, rather than *for*, the child
- ▲ Periodic reviews of the child's skills by the diabetes team
- ▲ A specific short-term plan for increasing and refining the child's skills
- ▲ Consistency of performance standards among the parents and the diabetes team

For adolescents and their parents, I often help negotiate an agreement that allows the adolescent to earn the parents' gradual withdrawal from involvement in specific diabetes tasks by showing lasting improvement in fulfilling that particular responsibility. One family agreed that if their teenaged daughter could show one month of consistent blood glucose testing with fewer than 25% of the results above 150 mg/dl, the parents would agree to look at her test results only once at the end of each month. Thus, both the teenager and the parents got something positive out of the situation.

Training Skills with Skill

The third characteristic for success is the parents' effectiveness as skill trainers and teachers. Children and adults learn in very different ways. Compared with adult learners, children are more dependent on getting hands-on experience, seeing many examples of the concepts being taught, breaking down complex skills into their components, and receiving immediate rewards for their efforts. Adults often overlook the fact that the many tasks that are expected of children and adolescents with diabetes are complicated. For example, correctly drawing up an insulin injection that contains a mixture of short-acting and intermediate-acting insulins requires perhaps two dozen distinct behavioral steps that must be completed in sequence.

Trying several different approaches to teaching different skills can help your child learn any task. For example, instead of simply demonstrating the skill, you might have your child talk you through each step in the skill sequence. You might also play a game in which your child's task is to identify errors in your technique as you demonstrate drawing up an insulin injection or performing a blood glucose test. The most complex skills can be broken down into segments and taught separately. For instance, you could draw up the first insulin type and then ask your child to draw up the second insulin type. The amount of physical guidance and verbal assistance that you offer can be withdrawn gradually until your child demonstrates competence with the skill in question. When teaching a young child to self-inject insulin, the parent could insert the needle and hold the barrel of the syringe in place while the child pushes down on the plunger. Then, gradually reduce the amount of help you give until your child is both holding the syringe and pushing down on the plunger. Next, move on to teaching the child to insert the needle. See Table 4-2 for some do's and don'ts for transferring diabetes responsibilities.

Table 4-2. **Do's and Don'ts of Transferring Diabetes Responsibility**

DO	DON'T
Ask your child how to solve diabetes problems instead of solving them yourself.	Immediately answer every question your child raises about diabetes.
Break down complex skills into a sequence of steps.	Expect perfect performance of complex skills.
Praise and reinforce effort and near misses.	Criticize failures or label your child as irresponsible.
Assume some responsibility for the child's self-management errors yourself.	Blame the child for all errors in self-management.
Step in when necessary to ensure your child's safety and to interrupt habitual errors or mistakes.	Tolerate recurring self-management errors by the child.
Teach all skills by gradually withdrawing physical assistance, verbal prompts, and supervision to maximize the child's success in gaining independence.	Abruptly expect that your child can complete a task correctly just by being told how to do it or just by having watched you do it.
Make sure that all adult caregivers and the diabetes team have the same definition of successful performance of the task in question.	Assume that everyone has the same standards for correct performance of each task.
React to failures and inconsistent performance from your child as natural parts of the learning process.	Blow your stack when your child makes a self-management error.
Ask your child how you can help.	Assume that you know how to help your child.
Communicate clearly and often with your child, your spouse, and your diabetes team about who is responsible for each aspect of diabetes treatment.	Assume that everyone agrees about who is responsible for each diabetes task.
Set specific short-term goals with your child to gradually increase his or her skills and independence.	Plod along with no specific short-term goals.

Talking About Complications:
Why, When, and How

There's another category of diabetes knowledge that children need to learn, one that's very difficult for many parents to teach—long-term complications. Yet, I still think that teaching about the long-term complications of diabetes is an important responsibility of parents and the health care team. Helping your preteen child understand the sources of your concern and fears may help you be clear about the goals of treatment, possibly reducing some of the common diabetes conflicts that happen between parents and teenagers. At the same time, communicating ineffectively about the long-term complications of diabetes can widen the generation gap considerably, so it's really important that this subject be approached in the right way. It's well-established that teens often have very incomplete or incorrect knowledge about a wide variety of health risks, such as those associated with tobacco, sexually transmitted diseases and sexual activity, and driving habits. It shouldn't be too surprising to learn that teens also tend to have misconceptions about the long-term heath risks that are posed by having diabetes. Yet, parents and health professionals often pull their hair out because teens seem to behave so irrationally with respect to these risks. Until you make sure that your child has accurate information about these risks, it's really not fair to judge their behavior in that way.

It's impossible to shelter youngsters with diabetes from learning that some people with diabetes face serious health risks years down the road. These facts, as well as many myths and misconceptions, will confront every youngster who in any way shows that he or she has diabetes. Even if children could be sheltered somehow from information (and misinformation) about the long-term complications of diabetes, I don't think that would be wise. By concealing the truth from kids, you're telling them, "I don't think you can handle it." This may lead them to either think that the situation is even worse than it really is or doubt their capacity to cope with it.

Helping your child learn about complications amounts, once again, to a process rather than an event. It's not very helpful to just give kids information and statistics about their risks for the various long-term complications of diabetes and leave it at that. There are some important factors to think about as you help your child through this process. Throughout childhood, your basic goal should be to help your child see that diabetes complications are something that you're comfortable talking about and that you're receptive to questions about. Try not to brush off your child's comments or questions because it makes you uncomfortable; view them instead as an invitation for further discussion. Using the threat of complications to try to motivate your youngster to be more responsible in diabetes self-care almost always does more harm than good; this usually only serves to discourage your child further. The risk of complications should only be discussed when you're calm and under control, not when you're angry with your child. Try to approach every discussion about complications with an optimistic perspective of prevention through healthy habits rather than in a threatening or ominous way.

All that young children really need to know is that it's important to keep their blood glucose under control to stay in the best possible health for the rest of their lives. Try to bring up this point now and then as a natural part of conversation. For example, when your third-grader tells you that he learned that smoking, overeating, and lack of exercise lead to heart attacks, you could let him know that, in a similar way, high blood glucose levels cause people with diabetes to have health problems as adults. It's not necessary to discuss specific complications with young children.

As children mature, their understanding of different organ systems increases, and they become capable of thinking about diseases in terms of multiple causes and interactions between risk factors. At this stage, it makes sense to begin giving children more detail about the specific health risks that they face.

Middle to late adolescents are generally capable of understanding most of the facts about long-term diabetes complications. At this point, I suggest giving your child reading material about complications or setting aside a specific time for your doctor or diabetes educator to discuss this topic with your teenager. If you find that it is too hard for you to assume these responsibilities, make sure that a doctor or nurse takes over for you.

For Fathers Only

Research has shown that mothers tend to shoulder most of the family's practical and emotional burdens that come along with raising a child who has diabetes. At the same time, kids from single-parent homes are known to fare more poorly when it comes to diabetic control and treatment adherence. Other research on healthy kids shows that the quality and quantity of a father's involvement are key factors that determine a wide variety of outcomes unrelated to diabetes, such as school performance, delinquency, peer relationships, substance abuse, and sexual activity. Kids fortunate enough to have fathers who are actively involved in their lives are likely to have better long-term outcomes on all of these issues. Why should coping with diabetes be any different? I am convinced that kids whose fathers are actively involved in their diabetes management are more cooperative with their treatment, have better emotional adjustment to having diabetes, and stay in better health. So how does a father's involvement produce these positive effects?

First, two sets of eyes and ears are better than one. When two adults are both actively informed and involved in the child's diabetes management, it is simply easier to effectively monitor treatment tasks, more immediate problem solving, and more frequent opportunities for encouragement and praise for the child's self-care behaviors. Second, the more fathers are involved, the less likely it is for mothers to "burn-out." Mothers who assume total responsibility for their child's diabetes management are likely to feel they have failed when things don't go well and frustrated if such problems persist or recur. Your interest, involvement, and encouragement may reduce or prevent these pitfalls, as well as help your child's mother to stick with it through some of the tough times. So, what can fathers, especially those with work responsibilities that get in the way, do to contribute effectively to their child's diabetes management? Here are some suggestions that are focused more on the quality, rather than the quantity, of your involvement:

▲ Ask your spouse at least once a week what you can do to help.

▲ Praise your spouse frequently both for her efforts in managing your child's diabetes and for her success in doing so.

▲ Talk about diabetes regularly with your child to show that you are informed, interested, and pleased about his or her self-management efforts.

▲ Exercise with your child regularly or support his/her involvement in organized sports.

▲ Adopt the same eating habits that are expected of your child with diabetes.

▲ Learn about diabetes by reading, attending workshops, using credible internet sources, etc.

TAKE-HOME MESSAGE

4 A proper balance of parent and child responsibilities for diabetes tasks aids the development of healthy self-management independence. Your child or teenager may be able to handle diabetes more effectively if you are able to stay involved in ways that are helpful and supportive.

MANAGING STRESS

Family Sharing of Diabetes Responsibilities

Family Communication

Emotional Coping

Diabetes Knowledge

Tameka was a 9-year-old girl who had been diagnosed with diabetes about three years earlier and had been doing very well and staying in very good diabetic control. Then for no obvious reason, her hemoglobin A1C results began going up sharply, and this continued even after several insulin adjustments and regular telephone calls from the diabetes nurse.

One day, Tameka's mother confided to a diabetes nurse that she had filed for divorce from her husband and that there had been a lot of fighting and arguing going on in the home. Once the divorce was final, and their situation calmed down, Tameka's diabetic control improved.

MANAGING STRESS

Everyone in today's world has to deal with stress in its many different forms. Stress can come from major life changes, like the death of a friend or relative, a divorce or separation, failing in school, wars, legal troubles, moving to a new home, or losing a job. Stress also comes in the form of daily hassles like driving in traffic, hectic schedules, too much homework, broken appliances, arguments, unexpected bills, and all of the other annoying experiences that we all must deal with every day. While we sometimes linger on the bad, positive changes in our lives like graduation, getting married, or receiving an award or promotion have the same kinds of physiological effects on our bodies as do these more negative experiences that we usually call stress.

It's a fact that stress can interfere with glucose control, and there are probably several ways in which this happens. All kinds of stress, whether from positive or negative experiences, can cause our bodies to release the so-called *stress hormones*—cortisol, growth hormone, and norepinephrine—that prepare us physically for either running away or doing battle. Back when we were cavemen, this feature came in very handy when we came face to face with a saber-toothed tiger in the forest. But we don't generally face life-threatening situations these days, so our bodies may be "over-equipped." This causes many of us to react too strongly when we face the kinds of stresses that exist in our modern world. Have you noticed any ways in which your body reacts (or maybe over-reacts) to psychological stress?

Although the stress hormones get us ready either to fight or to run away, they have another important effect when it comes to diabetes. These hormones also interfere with the action of insulin, causing blood glucose levels to increase. I'm sure our Neanderthal relatives wanted all the blood glucose they could muster when they were running away from that saber-toothed tiger. But, for us, experiencing psychological stress or not coping effectively with it can interfere directly with diabetic control by causing the release of stress hormones that block insulin and make it harder for insulin to work.

Stress can also interfere with diabetic control indirectly. When we are really stressed out, many of us naturally neglect our routine responsibilities in favor of focusing our energy on the sources of our stress. I'm sure you've noticed that, when you are under stress, your concentration, planning, and memory may not be as sharp as they usually are. Similarly, stress can also increase your child's risk of lapses in completing diabetes self-care responsibilities carefully or consistently enough. This can add to the direct physical effects of stress and result in poorer diabetic control.

Because nobody lives a stress-free life and stress can interfere with glucose control in several different ways, it is important that you and your child with diabetes learn to:

▲ Recognize the sources of stress impacting your family

▲ Understand the unique ways of coping with stress that exist in your family

▲ Develop a range of stress management skills or options that you can draw on in times of need

Can you think of times when stress seemed to interfere with your child's diabetic control?

Common Sources of Stress That May Interfere with Diabetic Control

Psychological stress is a very slippery concept. Some people seem to possess a hardiness or resilience that probably has its roots in early childhood. Such people may seem almost immune to the negative effects of stress. Others who lack these characteristics may collapse under the influence of even minor stresses and strains. Nonetheless, there are common stressful experiences that affect children and adolescents and that are generally expected to disrupt diabetic control:

▲ Family conflict, especially marital problems

▲ Separation and divorce and conflicts surrounding visitation or child support

▲ Stress related to work or school performance

▲ Friendships, romances, and pressure to engage in sexual activities

▲ Major losses such as death or unemployment

▲ Pressure to use drugs, alcohol, or tobacco

▲ Financial worries

▲ Dealing with the emotional side of diabetes

▲ Adjusting to others' reactions to diabetes

Does your child have any of these, or other, sources of psychological stress to deal with? If so, it would be valuable for you to consider how you can either reduce your child's exposure to that stress or help your child develop effective strategies for coping with it. And, if stresses like these are affecting your ability to help with your child's diabetes treatment, you should also be looking for ways to either reduce your stress level or to manage it more effectively.

Coping Styles: Different Strokes for Different Folks

Psychologists have written volumes in the past 25 years or so about how people seem to adopt characteristic "coping styles," which they tend to use when they're faced with stress, losses, or other psychological threats. Some people need to seek information about the sources of their stress. Others may distract themselves by becoming more involved in work or recreational interests. Some may have an intense need to share their experiences with others who have been through the same kind of stress. Others may switch into a problem-solving mode that drives them to seek a practical solution for removing or counteracting the stress. Of the different coping styles that have been described, the best coping style is simply the one that works for you. On the other hand, rigidly holding on to an ineffective or counterproductive coping style can be self-defeating and end up creating even more stress. You should also realize that different coping styles can clash. If an "information-seeker" happens to marry a "distracter," their differing coping styles can lead them to seek exactly the opposite kinds of relief. If that's the case in your family, try to give each other the space to use your own preferred coping methods and perhaps seek your own solitude through some mechanism outside of your family, such as the church, a support group, or another parent of a child with diabetes.

Effective Stress Management

There are countless effective ways to reduce or manage stress, ranging from just identifying stressful events to creating problem-solving strategies, enlisting social support, and gathering information. You, your child, and your spouse need to choose stress management strategies that are consistent with your most comfortable coping styles and that match the nature of the cause of your stress. People who are psychologically resilient and hardy are able to draw flexibly from a wide range of coping styles and strategies rather than having only a limited range of options. Most mental health professionals are experienced with helping people explore more effective stress management techniques. Perhaps your employer has an Employee Assistance Program with a plan geared toward stress relief. With these points in mind, here is a range of common stress management techniques that can be considered by children and adolescents with diabetes and their parents:

▲ Talk about your situation with a friend, neighbor, or relative. Try to find someone who has been through a similar problem. For further assistance, consider seeking help from a mental health professional.

▲ If you can't solve a problem, try to reframe or change the way you view it to make it less threatening or annoying.

▲ Break the problem down into smaller, more manageable parts. Sometimes by correcting part of a problem, what's left becomes more bearable.

▲ Make sure that you have realistic expectations for what you and your family can accomplish, both with respect to diabetes and in general.

▲ Give space to people who use different coping styles. Recognize that there are many different coping styles and techniques that can help people. When we stick rigidly to an ineffective coping style, we run into trouble.

▲ Identify, monitor, and change thought patterns that precede *feelings* of stress and anxiety. What you say to yourself about potentially stressful circumstances is probably more important than the circumstances themselves in determining whether you experience stress, anger, and anxiety.

▲ With the help of a mental health professional, learn progressive relaxation, transcendental meditation, yoga, or imagery techniques. Or try a stress management class offered by educational organizations, corporations, or hospitals to learn these skills and how to apply them to everyday stress.

▲ Look for ways to reduce the total demands on your time and energy. Eliminate unnecessary car trips, find more efficient ways to complete your errands, or figure out how to complete two or more routine tasks at the same time.

▲ Pay attention to your own needs for relaxation and fun. Spend time treating yourself to "healthy pleasures," like meditation, breathing fresh air, taking in sunshine, watching young children play, and enjoying nature.

▲ Adopt or buy a pet.

▲ Get 30 minutes of quiet solitude several times per week.

▲ Participate regularly in a diabetes support group. You can find these through your health care team. If there's not one in your area, see if you can find a health professional who will help you start one along with other families.

▲ Rely on spiritual support.

▲ Get regular physical exercise. Consistency is more important than intensity.

Compared to older children and adolescents, very young children may not show or express obvious negative reactions to family stress, which doesn't mean they are unaffected by it. Instead, young children might be more likely to have sleep or appetite problems, more dependence on their mothers, insecurity, strong habit patterns, and possibly aggressive or demanding behavior when they are facing stress. If you are the parent of a young child, when your family experiences stress I suggest that you consider the following approach. If your child probably isn't capable of understanding the stressful situation you are experiencing, discuss it away from the child. Be honest with your child about family stress and your feelings about it, but be careful not to overwhelm your child with more complex information than necessary. Answer your child's questions about the stress, being sure not to brush them off or dismiss them as silly. Don't put your child in the role of comforting you. When discussing the stress, try to relate the situation to something that your child has experienced previously and can remember. Try not to let family stress prevent you from setting appropriate limits and enforcing household rules for your child's behavior.

Caution: Don't Walk on Eggshells!

Even though stress can interfere with diabetic control, don't interpret this to mean that you should try to protect or shelter your child from experiencing psychological stress. Let's face it: your child is going to have to deal with plenty of stress in the future, and he or she needs to practice handling it while growing up. Don't make the mistake of thinking you can't impose rules, insist that chores be done, say no and mean it, or expect reasonable school performance from your child just because getting firm might raise your child's blood glucose. Parents who overindulge their children with diabetes as youngsters end up creating much more stress for themselves and their children in the future by raising a child who can't handle rules, tolerate limits, or delay gratification. Your child needs and wants discipline, so don't use stress reduction as an excuse for not giving it.

For Fathers Only

You and your partner may have plenty of reasons to be stressed out due to problems at work, finances, your relationships with each other or with other relatives, or any of hundreds of other big problems. Kids are a lot more sensitive than you might think to your stress level, and more importantly, the effectiveness of your coping ability. When your children see that you're having trouble coping, or that you respond to stress with anger, frustration, withdrawal, or the use of drugs or alcohol, you've taught them two bad lessons. One is that you've shown that life is overwhelming and the other is that you've provided an example of behaviors that your child really doesn't need to learn. Be part of the solution, not part of the problem. If you're caving into stress, that's nothing to be ashamed of— you have plenty of company. But your child needs you to find healthy and productive ways of responding to the challenges that life dishes out. Make that a priority and you may well find that the amount of stress in your life seems to drop way down. When you look closely at the causes of trouble in your life, the ripple effects of ineffective coping skills are often the source.

TAKE-HOME MESSAGE

5

Everyone experiences psychological stress that can potentially interfere with diabetic control. There are many effective styles and strategies that you can use for coping with stress, and you should help your youngster with diabetes develop a variety of flexible coping skills.

KEY

6

TREATMENT ADHERENCE

Managing Stress

Family Sharing of Diabetes Responsibilities

Family Communication

Emotional Coping

Diabetes Knowledge

Bethany, a 16 year-old girl, had developed type 1 diabetes nine years earlier. She lived with her parents and younger brother and sister. She was started on an insulin pump two years ago and at first she did very well. But in the past year, she had become less and less responsible about using it properly. She often forgot to give her insulin bolus until after she had eaten, rather than before the meal. Sometimes she gave her bolus without first checking her blood sugar. She often wrote down false blood sugar results in her logbook to avoid arguments with her mother. She frequently ate far more carbohydrates than her plan called for and usually didn't give more insulin when she did. Bethany and her parents had many arguments about her diabetes responsibilities and her mother asked the doctor if they should take her off the insulin pump.

Bethany's doctor referred the family to a psychologist who helped them to negotiate a behavioral contract through which Bethany could earn privileges that were important to her by fulfilling her doctor's expectations regarding blood sugar testing, insulin administration, and eating. Bethany remains on the insulin pump, she is more responsible about her diabetes, and she has a more positive and satisfying relationship with her parents and her doctor.

TREATMENT ADHERENCE

I'm fairly certain that the most common reason families of youngsters with diabetes seek the services of a psychologist or other mental health professional is trouble with *diabetes treatment adherence.* Adhering to an agreed-on treatment plan and meeting the treatment goals means that your child has to be consistent about carrying out the numerous treatment and self-monitoring tasks that go along with having diabetes. This is a challenge at any age—hence, the well-known problem of treatment adherence in adults with type 2 diabetes. Not sticking with treatment may be the most common cause of hospitalizations for poor diabetic control. It is also a major source of frustration and distress to health care professionals because it seems so difficult to understand. Additionally, there doesn't seem to be a simple one-to-one correspondence between treatment adherence and health outcomes in diabetes. Some children maintain very good diabetic control despite poor treatment adherence, whereas others have a hard time achieving acceptable diabetic control even with commendable adherence to their treatment plan.

This inconsistency between what most health professionals believe and many patients and families see as reality can set the stage for considerable frustration and friction. Some diabetes health care teams have begun adopting a "patient-empowerment" approach to this problem. Instead of a treatment relationship based on "Here is your treatment plan, now go and do it," more and more diabetes teams are approaching families from a different perspective: "How much are you willing to do to maintain your child's health and how can we help you to reach your goals?" Although this approach may be more satisfying to health professionals and to families, several key questions remain. Why is adequate treatment adherence so important? Why is it so hard to achieve? What can parents do to improve their youngster's treatment adherence?

As I've discussed, parents who stay involved in their children's diabetes management and make sure that the level of responsibility expected of the child is appropriate and guided carefully tend to see better treatment adherence. Family environments that are characterized by firm guidance, clearly stated rules, and frequent parental expressions of warmth and acceptance tend to have children who develop positive and healthy personal values. I'm sure that these same processes are at work in families of youngsters with diabetes and that they influence whether the child accepts the responsibilities of diabetes as something they want to do for themselves or whether they reject those responsibilities as something that has been imposed on them by unreasonable adults.

Why Treatment Adherence Is So Important

Researchers have worked for decades to study the relationship between treatment adherence and diabetic control, and I'll try to briefly summarize all of that work here. The Diabetes Control and Complications Trial (DCCT) proved that maintaining near-normal blood glucose levels over time prevents or reduces the long-term complications of diabetes, including damage to the eyes, kidneys, blood vessels, and nerves. Poor adherence with the treatment plan may prevent people with diabetes from achieving the best possible diabetic control, which increases the risk of future long-term diabetic complications.

Poor adherence seems to be the most common reason for hospitalizations and emergency room visits for diabetic ketoacidosis and severe hypoglycemia. Most youngsters who are admitted to the hospital can be quickly restored to good glucose control if their insulin treatments and meal plan are carried out carefully under supervised conditions. In other words, most hospitalizations of children and adolescents with diabetes are preventable. The worse the treatment adherence, the more difficult it becomes for the diabetes health care team to make sure that the prescribed treatment plan is the most appropriate one for the person with diabetes.

So, poor adherence has the potential for damaging your child's health. In addition, not following the prescribed diabetes treatment plan hurts relationships. Poor adherence is a common source of conflicts and arguments between teenagers with diabetes and their parents. Poor adherence can also inhibit a trusting relationship between the family and the health care team. And so, even if there is not a simple, one-to-one relationship between treatment adherence and diabetic control, acceptable adherence is still a worthwhile goal.

Despite these compelling arguments, few patients and families achieve excellent adherence consistently over long periods. In fact, almost no patients in the DCCT were able to do this, despite the fact that they were pre-selected as "model" patients at the beginning of the study. This isn't unique to diabetes either; it's true of just about every chronic medical condition, and it happens among people of all ages and income levels. The reasons for this have their roots in some basic principles that govern our behavior.

Why Treatment Adherence Is So Hard

Just as there are many good reasons why carrying out the treatment plan as prescribed makes a lot of sense, there are plenty of explanations why so many youngsters, especially teens, have a lot of trouble doing this.

▲ Taking good care of diabetes requires time and energy that many youngsters would rather devote to other activities.

▲ Many kids think that much of diabetes treatment either hurts or deprives them of desired foods, drinks, or activities.

▲ Performing treatment or monitoring tasks may serve as a reminder of one's illness and an indication of being different from others.

▲ Diabetes treatment may conflict with youngsters' goals regarding their body weight. Good diabetic control and healthy nutrition may cause weight gain that many kids, especially girls, would rather avoid. Concerns about weight gain may lead some adolescents to eat less or to take less insulin to try to lose weight.

▲ Occasional lapses in treatment adherence don't usually lead immediately and directly to bad consequences. Compared with parents and health professionals, it is normal for children and adolescents to be much less concerned about the long-term consequences of their behavior, including the prospects of poor diabetic control. Instead, they are focused on the present and immediate future. These differences in perspective have the net effect of ensuring that good treatment adherence is more important to adults than to the child or adolescent with diabetes.

▲ Blood glucose testing often yields bad news and may precipitate more conflict with parents than simply not testing.

▲ Fear of hypoglycemia may cause some children to overeat and keep their blood glucose levels a little high to prevent hypoglycemic reactions.

▲ Diabetes treatment offers adolescents a convenient platform for asserting their independence and for demonstrating their bravery and invincibility through risk-taking behavior.

▲ Our zeal in encouraging self-management of diabetes may create the impression that poor diabetic control is always and only a failure of self-management and that blame rests only with the child. Many youngsters view themselves as failures and become very discouraged about their chances for good diabetic control.

You probably thought about many of these points yourself, but seeing them all in one long list may make it easier to understand why it's so difficult for many youngsters to keep up with all that diabetes asks of them. When I look over this list, it surprises me that so many young people do a really good job of keeping up with all of the responsibilities imposed on them by diabetes.

How You Can Influence Treatment Adherence

Every science has its own collection of laws—basic principles that are so well established that they have become widely accepted as facts. In psychology, we have what we call the Law of Effect. In short, this law states that behavior followed by positive reinforcement tends to be repeated and behavior followed by punishment tends to decrease in strength. The flip side of this law is that behaviors that result in the loss or withdrawal of reinforcement will decrease, whereas behaviors that work to escape or avoid punishment will increase. And so, there are two basic ways to increase a behavior: you can either deliver positive reinforcement or remove punishment. By the same token, there are two ways to decrease a behavior: you can either deliver punishment or remove reinforcement.

I favor positive reinforcement for desired behaviors over the other three possible behavior change strategies. I think that living with diabetes is unpleasant enough without making self-care a focus for even more negative interactions and disappointments. I believe in allowing youngsters with diabetes to earn small, frequent tokens of positive reinforcement by fulfilling the self-care responsibilities that are expected of them. I don't see any difference between this approach and letting kids earn a part of their weekly allowance by doing household chores or giving them a bonus for As or Bs on their report cards. I don't believe that you spoil kids by having them earn something they value by meeting agreed-on goals. Is your boss spoiling you by giving you a paycheck or by handing out a bonus if you exceed your performance goals? Sure, your other children may ask for the same kind of treatment, and I think that's a good sign. It's like them saying, "I want to be good, too, and I want you to help me do it!" Refusing to use positive reinforcement is like tying one hand behind your back as a parent because it means that you're not putting a basic law of behavior totally to work for you. When used correctly, positive reinforcement is the strongest tool that parents have to encourage good treatment adherence.

Why Poor Treatment Adherence Occurs

In the past few decades, much has been learned about treatment adherence in general and adherence to diabetes therapy specifically. One fact about treatment adherence is that it tends to decline with age during childhood. It often becomes a significant problem during the teenage years. Among the many reasons for this is the fact that adolescents develop a physiological resistance to insulin, which means they need a larger dose per pound of body weight than at any other time in their lives. This may make it a little harder to control their blood glucose levels. This can be discouraging to the teenager who has coasted through the late childhood years with near-normal blood glucose. Rebellion, risk taking, and fierce individualism are all common during the teen years, and these features don't mesh well with some of the requirements of diabetes treatment. Teens place a high priority on gaining the acceptance of friends and classmates by conforming to current trends, so appearing different from the peer group is threatening. The diabetes regimen also places a premium on consistency, organization, and foresight, which are characteristics that are often not well-developed in teenagers. Sometimes it's hard for parents and health professionals to realize that adolescents aren't yet adults psychologically. Sure, their bodies may be full grown and they may be able to hold their own in arguments with their parents, but they are going to need a few more years of patient guidance and limit setting before they reach adult levels of maturity in areas such as personal responsibility, organization, planning, and delaying gratification. There are still plenty of things that you can do to smooth things out during this challenging period.

Just as adolescents vary greatly in terms of their personalities, talents, and habits, so do families. Much research has been aimed at determining which characteristics of families are associated with treatment adherence. Remember, parents who are more involved in the child's diabetes management tend to have youngsters with better treatment adherence and diabetic control. Direct and honest family communication and effective conflict resolution skills also seem to produce better diabetes outcomes. Families who support and reward good adherence rather than emphasizing punishment and criticism for poor adherence achieve better results. Children tend to internalize important values when they are raised in an environment characterized by warmth, acceptance, and consistent limits. These same processes probably determine whether children with diabetes adopt positive values about their health care. Finally, families with clearly defined responsibilities and expectations for what is to be done—when, how often, and by whom—achieve the most consistent treatment adherence.

There are several ways in which what a youngster does to take care of his or her diabetes might differ from what was intended by the diabetes team. These differences occur for a range of reasons and therefore require specialized responses from parents and the diabetes health care team.

▲ Some youngsters might not do as expected because they don't know what is expected, they don't have the skill needed to fulfill the expectation, or they don't have the necessary supplies or equipment. In any of these situations, a more thorough assessment of the child's circumstances by the physician or diabetes educator usually leads directly to an appropriate solution. It's a good idea to rule out these kinds of barriers before jumping on your teenager with both feet.

▲ Some adolescents may intentionally subvert the diabetes regimen by skipping insulin doses or eating large quantities of sweets, often in an attempt to communicate, however indirectly, some unresolved emotional turmoil or interpersonal conflict. In these cases, a mental health professional almost certainly needs to be involved.

▲ Some very young children with diabetes may be unable to tolerate the pain involved with insulin injections and blood glucose tests.

▲ Because children focus on internal cues when deciding to eat, they may be inconsistent eaters.

▲ Older children and adolescents may have all the skills they need to do what is expected of them, but lack the organization, memory, sense of responsibility, or motivation necessary to get the job done.

In my experience, this last problem is the most common type of adherence problem, and it may require calling on a mental health professional. There are some steps you can take before you should start looking for a psychologist or psychiatrist.

How to Improve Treatment Adherence

Toddlers, Preschoolers, and Young Children

Some very young children with diabetes show a lot of fear and resistance when it's time for insulin injections and blood glucose tests. They may run, hide, throw temper tantrums, and otherwise make life miserable for their already guilt-ridden and overwrought parents. Although most parents eventually get the job done, it's a major challenge that can be emotionally draining. Here are a few ideas about how to minimize these problems:

▲ Give your child some control over the situation by offering choices regarding which finger to stick, which site to use for insulin injections, or which parent will do the deed. These can all be negotiable, but the tasks still have to be carried out.

▲ Prepare the materials for the blood glucose test and injections away from the child's view, if at all possible. When it's time, go and bring the child to where the test and injection will be done rather than calling the child to come to you.

▲ Teach your child to focus on some object just before the procedure, and coach the child in using controlled breathing to stay calm. One approach that captures the attention of many young children is to have them blow a party horn or a pinwheel or blow up a balloon during the procedure.

▲ Explain to your child that the doctors and nurses want you to do these things to keep him or her as healthy as possible.

▲ Give lots of praise after any evidence of an improved reaction to the procedure. Also, emphasize to your child realistically that both procedures hurt a little but only for an instant.

▲ Keep on hand a grab bag of small toys or trinkets and allow your child to reach in for a surprise after showing acceptable cooperation with the procedures. Kids are constantly asking for small treats in supermarkets and discount stores. I encourage you to pick up some of these to stock your grab bag, and allow your child to earn them later.

Eating problems are also common among very young children with diabetes. These problems include extreme pickiness about the foods that are served, dawdling, and insisting that mom make something else. Some kids can be unpredictable about what, when, and how much they will eat. Here are a few ideas to help you encourage better eating by your child:

▲ Your goals should be to convince your child that his or her eating is not very important to you and to avoid letting it become a battleground.

▲ If your child's pre-meal blood glucose was above 120 mg/dl, it may not be critical that the child eat right now.

▲ Give your child the opportunity to choose what you will prepare or serve from among several available food choices. Offer these choices only before the meal, never once the meal has been pre-pared and served.

▲ You may want to restrict snacks to within 60 to 90 minutes before meals and wait to offer the meal until your child reports being hungry.

▲ The grab-bag approach can also be used to encourage more reli-able eating and appropriate mealtime behavior.

▲ When your child eats with other children, praise the good eating behavior of other children at the table.

▲ Consider offering four or five "mini-meals" per day to your child. Many young children are overwhelmed by seeing a large amount of food on a plate, so putting less food on the plate may help them feel that eating the meal is possible.

▲ In general, devote much more effort to praising any and all hints of appropriate eating and other mealtime behaviors rather than begging, cajoling, and pleading with your child to eat. I don't rec-ommend catering to children who refuse to eat by running to the kitchen to prepare them something other than what you have made.

▲ If your child is taking you down the primrose path by refusing to eat, you might try to end the meal after a reasonable period, say 20 minutes, but then do a blood glucose test every 15 to 20 minutes until the child chooses to eat. This may seem a little brutal, but it is a logical natural consequence that is necessary to preserve your child's safety if the pre-meal insulin has been given. Some diabetes teams might allow some parents of poor or unpredictable eaters to defer giving the pre-meal insulin until after the child eats. The recent introduction of very fast acting insulins provides another alternative that may be used in this circumstance. Discuss these options with your child's doctor or diabetes team.

Older Children and Adolescents

Older children and adolescents present very different kinds of problems in fulfilling their diabetes self-care responsibilities, and they require a different approach. In general, the effectiveness of any intervention to promote treatment adherence among adolescents depends a great deal on whether the teenager perceives the approach as pushy or supportive. Adolescents who feel pushed can be expected to push back, which usually means worse treatment adherence or derailing the treatment plan in some other, less obvious way. The concept of patient empowerment, which places the patient at the center of the health care team, has become increasingly accepted by diabetes educators in the past few years. Helping adolescents feel empowered and less imposed upon can help lower some of the typical resistance to guidance and suggestions offered by adults. A good first step to dealing with poor treatment adherence in an adolescent is to try to empower the youngster by asking:

▲ What part of living with diabetes is the most difficult or unsatisfying for you?

▲ How does this situation make you feel?

▲ How does it interfere with your personal goals?

▲ How would this situation have to change for you to feel better about it?

▲ Are you willing to take action to improve the situation for yourself?

▲ What steps could you take to bring you closer to where you want to be?

▲ Is there one thing that you will do from now on to improve things for you?

A second important concept that will help your adolescent improve his or her self-care responsibility is a willingness to compromise and to work gradually toward a goal by starting where the teenager is right now. Adolescents can be easily overwhelmed and discouraged about the prospect of striving toward a major long-term behavior change goal. They will often cooperate much more readily with parents who are willing to accept gradual, stepwise change toward an intermediate goal rather than insisting on perfect self-care immediately. Expecting perfect performance of a self-care behavior that has been happening only 10% of the time for the past 6 months is doomed to fail.

The most common adherence problems during adolescence tend to involve failing to accept responsibility for blood glucose testing, poor eating choices, skipping insulin doses, unreliable recording of self-monitoring and insulin data, and not waiting to eat after taking insulin. Here are some practical things you can do to help your older child or adolescent carry out these diabetes self-care behaviors as consistently as possible:

▲ Make sure that you, your child, and the health care team have the same ideas about what is expected and how often and who is responsible for each part of the treatment plan. It's common for this simple first step to be overlooked.

▲ Look for opportunities to praise and reward good self-care. Try to do this much more often than punishing or criticizing self-care failures or shortcomings. A little acknowledgment can go a long way with most children.

▲ Talk openly with your health care team about any treatment expectations that have been particularly difficult to carry out consistently. Your team may be able to suggest modified plans or compromises that haven't yet been tried.

▲ Negotiate with your teen to establish reasonable and achievable intermediate goals rather than expecting immediate perfect performance. For example, if your teenaged son is completing only 30% of his blood glucose tests, you could allow him to earn a reward by completing 50% over the next two weeks. When he succeeds at that, then you could increase the target to 70% for a few weeks, and so on.

▲ Have frequent family meetings and include diabetes self-care on the agenda at every meeting. (See Key #3.)

▲ Expect and plan for times when adherence will be difficult. Give your child permission to tell you when "it's all too much" and that he or she needs extra help in getting the job done.

▲ Use nonverbal cues, such as calendars, signs, or pictures, instead of coaxing, prodding, or nagging to get kids to fulfill their self-care responsibilities. One family came up with the idea of taping two new insulin syringes to the refrigerator door each morning that their daughter would then use for her injections. This provided an easy way to see if she had given her insulin and minimized the need for nagging and reminding.

▲ Rotate responsibilities between the parents for supervising and encouraging the child's diabetes adherence. Be clear about which parent is on duty, and trade off at regular intervals.

▲ Enlist "helper" adults who can support your child in making healthy self-care choices in school and other settings away from home. For example, there may be a teacher or other staff member in your child's school who is familiar with diabetes, or willing to learn about it, who could help your child make healthy food choices for lunch.

▲ Avoid letting diabetes become entangled in other family problems like conflicts between separated or divorced parents over the child's glucose control. Teenagers understandably resent being the focus of intense conflicts between their parents and will sometimes undermine the diabetes regimen as a way of expressing their anger.

▲ Ask your doctor for a referral to mental health professional if your child's treatment adherence has been a consistent problem for three to six months and either your child's A1C has increased significantly or more than one emergency room visit or hospital-ization has been necessary.

One tool that works effectively to support positive changes in diabetes self-care behaviors is the *behavioral contract*. A behavioral contract is a written agreement that allows the child to earn small, weekly rewards or privileges by fulfilling verified treatment and test-ing requirements. Effective behavioral contracts are based on gen-uine negotiation. In negotiating a behavioral contract, parents and teens:

▲ Decide on a clearly defined target or goal

▲ Choose measurable short-term objectives

▲ Establish methods of verifying progress toward the objectives

▲ Arrange for frequent positive consequences for meeting the terms of the contract

▲ Specify dates and times for evaluation and re-negotiation of the contract

Be careful about negotiating behavioral contracts that target improved *diabetic control* rather than improved behavioral changes. If improving glucose control is something you feel should be the overall objective, be sure to set realistic short-term goals. For exam-ple, if 60% of your daughter's test results in the past month have been below 180 mg/dl, it makes little sense to expect that she can improve immediately to 100% of test results below 180 mg/dl. Instead, reward her for reaching an intermediate goal, perhaps low-ering her blood glucose so that 75% of her results are below 180 mg/dl. Once she's achieved success at that level for at least a month, then think about encouraging her to go after even better control. In my experience, many parents and health care professionals expect youngsters to demonstrate too much improvement too quickly, and this unrealistic expectation is probably the most common reason for failure when this method doesn't work. Look at the following sample contracts for some ideas on what's appropriate for these ele-ments of the contract.

SAMPLE BEHAVIORAL CONTRACT #1

Eric, 12 years old

Child: Eric Johnson   *Date:* July 31, 2003
Parents: William & Denise Johnson   *Physician:* B. Donovan, MD
Problem Targeted for Improvement:

Not doing enough blood glucose tests.

Problem Definition: Eric has completed an average of 0.8 tests per day over the last two months. He often gives himself insulin injections without having done a blood glucose test.

Behavioral Objective: Eric will average completing two blood glucose tests per day over the next two weeks.

Method of Monitoring: Mr. Johnson will check the memory of Eric's meter every Sunday night at bedtime.

Consequences: Eric will earn packages of football cards for meeting the behavioral objectives of this contract as follows:

- If his meter shows that he has done fewer than 28 tests in the past two weeks, he will earn no football cards.

- If his meter shows that he has done 28 to 41 tests in the past two weeks, he will earn one package of football cards.

- If his meter shows that he has done 42 to 55 tests in the past two weeks, he will earn three packages of football cards.

- If his meter shows that he has done 56 or more tests in the past two weeks, he will earn six packages of football cards.

Evaluation Date: August 15, 2003

Signed _____   Signed _____
             PARENT   PARENT

Signed _____
             CHILD

SAMPLE BEHAVIORAL CONTRACT #2

Blake, 17 years old

Child: Blake Martin   *Date: August* 1, 2003
Parents: James & Vera Martin   *Physician:* R. Thompson, MD
Problem Targeted for Improvement:

**Overeating; eating off schedule; taking extra insulin
without telling parents or testing blood glucose first.**

Problem Definition: According to his dietitian, Blake has averaged about 115 grams of carbohydrate per day recently. His meal plan allows 100 grams of carbohydrate. His blood glucose has averaged 238 mg/dl over the past month. He admits that he takes a few extra units of Regular insulin two or three times per week when he feels like eating a heavy snack.

Behavioral Objectives: 1) Blake will reduce his average blood glucose level to 180 mg/dl for the next two weeks. 2) Blake will record his carbohydrate intake and insulin use daily for the next two weeks. 3) Blake will see a psychologist weekly for help with getting these problems under control.

Method of Monitoring: Mrs. Martin will review the blood glucose tests recorded in Blake's meter once per week on Sunday nights and will record the average blood glucose for the two-week period. Mr. Martin will examine Blake's records of carbohydrate intake and insulin use at bedtime each night, and he will prompt Blake to record this information as it happens.

Consequences: Blake will receive $5 allowance per week, and he will have the chance to earn a total allowance bonus of $15 by meeting the behavioral objectives outlined above. For each of the objectives that he fulfills in any two-week period, he will receive a bonus of $5.

Evaluation Date: September 15, 2003

Signed _____   Signed _____
       PARENT   PARENT

Signed _____
       CHILD

SAMPLE BEHAVIORAL CONTRACT #3

Rachel, 14 years old

Child: Rachel Gomez   *Date:* August 1, 2003
Parents: Eduardo & Vera Gomez   *Physician:* W. Tuttle, M.D.
Problem Targeted for Improvement:

Weight control.

Problem Definition: Rachel weighs 273 pounds (112 kilograms), compared with an ideal body weight of 126 pounds (57 kilograms). Her physicians states that she has a good chance of staying off insulin for treatment of type 2 diabetes if she can lose at least 100 pounds.

Behavioral Objectives: 1) Rachel will record her calorie intake after each meal. 2) Rachel will limit her calorie intake to no more than 2,200 calories per day and will attempt to lose three pounds every two weeks. 3) Rachel will limit her time on the computer, playing video games, or watching TV to one hour per day. She will play or exercise outdoors at least two hours per day.

Method of Monitoring: Mrs. Gomez will check Rachel's records of her calorie intake at random intervals at least three times per week. Mrs. Gomez will ensure that Rachel uses the computer, TV, and video game equipment for no more than one hour daily and that she goes outside for play or exercise at least two hours daily. Mr. Gomez will exercise with Rachel at least 30 minutes daily during the week and at least one hour daily on weekends and holidays. Mrs. Gomez will take Rachel to her doctor's office once each two weeks to weigh in and she will record the weight as measured by the clinic nurse.

Consequences: Rachel will be allowed to avoid babysitting her younger brother if she meets her weight loss goal of three pounds every two weeks. Rachel will earn $1 each time her mother checks her calorie record book and finds that it is up to date. Rachel will earn $1 for each day that she meets her goals of less than one hour using the computer, TV, or video games and at least two hours of outdoor play and/or exercise.

Evaluation Date: September 15, 2003

Signed _____   Signed _____
      PARENT   PARENT

Signed _____
      CHILD

TAKE-HOME MESSAGE

6

Perfect treatment adherence is a praiseworthy goal, but few patients and their families achieve it consistently, and there isn't always a simple one-to-one relationship between adherence and diabetic control. It's important that you keep lines of communication open, anticipate lapses as a natural part of life with diabetes, and focus much more effort on positive reinforcement of good self-care behaviors rather than on punishment and criticism for self-care failures.

DIABETES PROBLEM SOLVING

Treatment Adherence

Managing Stress

Family Sharing of Diabetes Responsibilities

Family Communication

Emotional Coping

Diabetes Knowledge

Jeremy was diagnosed with type 1 diabetes at 12 years of age and for the past 3 years he had never really been in good control of his diabetes. Even though he tested his blood sugar frequently, neither he nor his mother seemed to know what they could do to correct his usually high blood sugars. Using a computer to analyze his blood glucose profile, a diabetes educator found that Jeremy's results were often high in the morning and that his results tended to stay high whenever that was the case. So, she helped Jeremy and his mother to learn how to recognize this pattern and she helped them to make an adjustment to the carbohydrate content of his bedtime snack and to his bedtime insulin dosage. He has maintained much better diabetic control since making those changes. He and his mother have also shown a lot more interest in learning other problem-solving strategies.

DIABETES PROBLEM SOLVING

Everyone with diabetes, whether a child, adolescent, or adult, will encounter roadblocks now and then, despite doing everything they can to stay on top of their diabetes self-care responsibilities. Those who aren't so careful may find that dealing with these unexpected challenges is much more difficult, maybe resulting in more frequent severe hypoglycemia, hospitalizations, and emergency room visits. On the other hand, living well with diabetes is basically the same thing as knowing how to anticipate and solve the many problems that it can pose every day. Living with diabetes on a day-to-day basis means that you and your child will be faced with countless situations like these:

▲ Without announcing it in advance, the school cafeteria changes the lunch schedule so that your son will be eating 45 minutes later than before.

▲ Your daughter's blood glucose levels before supper have been above 220 mg/dl for 5 of the past 7 days.

▲ Your son has been on the track team, but he sprained his ankle and will be unable to run for 2 weeks.

▲ Your child has a fever, vomiting, and diarrhea and can't keep anything down.

▲ Your son will soon be going on his first overnight trip with the school basketball team.

▲ Your family will be flying to visit relatives three time zones away, and you're not sure how to change your child's insulin schedule.

▲ Your teenager works three afternoons a week, and on those days, she eats dinner 3 hours later than on the other days of the week.

▲ A few minutes after your daughter took her insulin and you ordered dinner for her, the waiter returns to tell you that her order was ruined and the cook will have to start over.

▲ Your son has joined a soccer team that practices for 2 hours each afternoon on Mondays, Wednesdays, and Saturdays, but not at all on the other days.

Sound familiar? When I've asked parents and youngsters with diabetes to tell me the hardest part of living with diabetes, one of the most common answers is that it is always there and it never goes away. Situations like those I listed above are probably a major source of that feeling.

Having diabetes complicates your life and brings up problems that probably weren't solved for you in the diabetes textbooks that you've read. These problems can be stressful, frustrating, and scary, and they often require you to think quickly on your feet. At the same time, though, they provide you with several important opportunities. Problems like those above offer a chance to teach your child about more sophisticated diabetes self-management skills and to shape a self-confident attitude toward diabetes. They can give you and your child valuable practice fitting diabetes flexibly into your family's lifestyle rather than changing your lifestyle to suit diabetes. They provide a way to show your child that blood glucose tests have a purpose beyond simply being reviewed by a doctor or nurse every few months, which may also increase your child's willingness to test. They give you a chance to strengthen your position as an expert on your child's diabetes. They offer a way to teach your child how to make the most effective use of the health care team as a consultant in situations that require problem solving. When you look at problems as opportunities, the hurdles that diabetes places in your path actually give you and your family the chance to become "empowered" over diabetes, to lay claim to a primary role at the center of the diabetes treatment team. This is a way to gain a measure of freedom from the feeling that diabetes is oppressive and the fact that it never goes away. In the Diabetes Control and Complications Trial (DCCT), patients who learned, by trial and error, to solve problems by adjusting their diabetes treatment regimen had the best success in achieving and maintaining near-normal blood glucose levels. In effect, they learned to control their diabetes rather than letting their diabetes control them. You and your child can learn to do the same if you're able to commit some time and effort.

Diabetes Problems or Opportunities?

Why is it so important to give yourself and your child diabetes problem-solving tools and practice? Because diabetes is there all the time, every day. Most children and adolescents with diabetes spend only an hour or so every few months with their diabetes team, perhaps with a few telephone calls every once in a while. The other 99% of their time is spent with their family and friends and in school. Time away from home increases steadily throughout childhood. Obviously, this is where diabetic control does or does not happen. Many of the day-to-day issues that arise regarding diabetes treatment are most effectively addressed quickly and decisively rather than waiting for the chance to reach a doctor or nurse by telephone.

There are plenty of tools that can help you learn diabetes problem solving (see the "Resources" section). It is important for you to learn these skills. "Outsmarting" diabetes puts you in the driver's seat instead of just going along for the ride. Being in charge, however, requires that:

▲ Your knowledge of diabetes be sound

▲ You and your child keep glucose control a high priority

▲ You view yourselves as the center of the diabetes team

▲ You have enough self-confidence to think on your feet in order to solve daily diabetes problems

I'm advocating a substantial investment of time and energy on your part, but it's one that often pays off handsomely.

It's natural in the early months of dealing with their children's diabetes that parents are too involved learning the basics about diabetes to consider fine-tuning diabetic control. Even after some hands-on experience with managing diabetes on a day-to-day basis, the notion of taking a larger, decision-making role in evaluating and adjusting the treatment regimen might seem threatening. First, your family needs to get used to the daily rigors of diabetes self-care and you and your child need experience working with your health care team to analyze and resolve a range of typical problems. The next natural step is to anticipate or even suggest actions that you need to take as problems occur. As your confidence, skills, and experience grow, you may find that when you call for help or advice a diabetes team member will ask you what the most appropriate solution for you would be. When you've reached that stage, it's time for you to begin teaching your child to become a self-confident diabetes problem-solver.

A Family Problem-Solving System

One way for parents to develop solid diabetes problem-solving skills, and help their children learn these skills, is to get in the habit of using a systematic, structured approach to group problem solving. Below is a step-by-step method for group problem solving that has been tested in lots of other situations like marriage counseling, labor relations, and quality-improvement programs in many businesses. This approach works well for those hassles and disappointments that seem to happen again and again, and it can be applied just as easily to recurring problems with managing diabetes. If you're trying this approach for the first time, you should choose a minor, low-conflict issue to discuss. If you're successful with that one, then take on something a little more challenging the next time. This system fits nicely into the framework for family meetings that I outlined in Key #3. Here are the six steps that make up this system:

1. **Problem definition:** Each family member should be given the opportunity to define the problem in his or her own words. It may be necessary to break down the problem into several smaller problems and address each one separately. Write down the defi-

nition of the problem that you've selected to work on together. *Example:* Jessica's blood glucose before supper on school days has averaged 226 mg/dl over the past 3 weeks, but it has averaged 142 over the same period on weekends.

2. **Verification:** Make sure that each family member agrees with the problem's definition. Give everyone a chance to define the problem in their own words and to get feedback from the other family members. Continue revising the definition until everyone is okay with it.

3. **Brainstorming:** Without interruption, each family member should be allowed to suggest possible solutions to the selected problem. The emphasis in this step should be on free and creative thinking and on generating lots of ideas. Try to come up with 8 to 10 possible solutions, and write them down. Family members should refrain from evaluating one another's suggestions during this step.

Examples:

▲ Jessica should eat a smaller snack after school

▲ Parents should call her doctor about increasing the morning insulin dose

▲ Jessica should delay eating supper until her blood glucose is less than 120 mg/dl

▲ Jessica should be rewarded if she lowers her blood glucose before supper on school days

▲ Jessica should take a bike ride or play softball after school

▲ Jessica should join an after-school activity to keep her busy

▲ Jessica should walk home from school or ride her bike instead of being driven home

▲ Parents should test Jessica's blood glucose when she returns home from school and plan her snack according to the result

4. **Evaluation of solutions:** This is the time for each family member to consider each suggested solution, discuss any potential barriers to carrying it out, and evaluate the likely effects of the solution on the selected problem. It's a good idea to let each family

member rate each solution as positive (likely to be effective) or negative (not likely to be effective).

5. **Action plan:** Now try to develop a plan of attack by selecting from among your positively rated solutions. Write down the goal of your action plan. Look for opportunities to combine solutions or to come up with compromises. Your action plan should specify clearly what will be done, who will do it, when it will be done, and how it will be evaluated. Make sure that everyone agrees to the action plan and that possible barriers to it being carried out have been anticipated and dealt with satisfactorily.
Example: The goal is to reduce Jessica's average blood glucose at suppertime to 140 mg/dl every day of the week. The parents will test Jessica's blood glucose when she gets home from school and plan her snack accordingly. Jessica will ride her bike to and from school instead of having her mother drive her to school. Jessica will earn $3 for each week that her blood glucose averages less than 140 mg/dl before supper for the week.

6. **Evaluation and refinement of solution:** Set a date and time when you will get together again to reevaluate the action plan. If the goal wasn't met, go back to Step 1 above, and try to figure out how the problem definition or action plan could be changed or refined to increase its effectiveness. Keep doing this until you're satisfied that the problem has been solved, and then move on to another problem.
Example: The family will meet again in 4 weeks to see if the goal was met. It will be evaluated by looking at Jessica's pre-supper blood glucose test results that are stored in the memory of her glucose meter.

This approach works well for those pesky problems that seem to happen again and again. But you and your youngster also need to be prepared to think on your feet, to anticipate and solve the kinds of diabetes problems that just seem to come up without warning. At those times, you won't always have the benefit of a calm and thoughtful group discussion about your options. Effective diabetes problem-solving of this type requires a lot of confidence in your knowledge and skills, plenty of experience with your child's diabetes, and a lot of creative thinking. These aren't easy skills to come by, but the effort you put into developing them can pay off immensely in giving you and your child a great deal more freedom and a sense of greater control over your daily lives.

How to Become a Diabetes Problem Solver

There have been few research studies of this crucial part of diabetes self-care, despite its obvious importance to diabetic control and quality of life. The studies that have been done tend to suggest that families of children with diabetes use their blood glucose data infrequently to adjust insulin, food, or exercise to keep blood glucose levels near normal. The most common use of blood glucose data in one study was in managing low blood glucose levels. Much less common uses of blood glucose data were to prevent problems that are anticipated but had yet to occur. Families that frequently used blood glucose test results for treatment adjustments generally had better parental knowledge of diabetes, less family conflict, and better overall adherence with the medical regimen. In other words, many families could be making more effective use of blood glucose test results.

Here are some practical suggestions to help you become an expert diabetes problem solver and train your child to do the same.

▲ Be on the lookout every day for those little events that pose a "diabetes problem," a situation in which reaching a solution would be of immediate value or interest to you. This is what educators call a "teachable moment." Keep a diary in which you note the problem, your solution, and the outcome.

▲ Seek out more advanced diabetes education.

▲ Learn how to identify patterns in your child's blood glucose profile, how to adjust insulin doses in response to the patterns you've identified, and how to adjust insulin, the meal plan, or exercise for expected changes in your child's routine. Ask your physician and diabetes educator to describe their philosophy and help you develop these skills.

▲ Develop a systematic approach to reviewing your child's blood glucose results, aimed more at detecting and understanding patterns than at trying to understand individual test results.

▲ Try to avoid tunnel vision. Instead of worrying about a single test result, look for patterns and consistencies over a series of test results. Keep your frame of reference in terms of days and weeks rather than minutes or hours.

▲ Look for any regularity in the times or days when the most extreme test results have occurred. For example, you may find that your child's blood glucose is often high in the morning before breakfast and that, when it is, you have a hard time getting it back down the rest of that day. If you were to call your clinic with that type of observation, your doctor or nurse could probably help you adjust your child's evening insulin dose to prevent the high blood glucose levels in the mornings.

▲ Have brainstorming sessions with your child and other family members shortly before scheduled clinic visits to come up with ideas for improving or stabilizing diabetic control. Then you will be prepared to discuss your ideas with the health care team. The emphasis here should be on generating a large number of ideas and looking for creative ways to combine some of them.

▲ With your child and diabetes care team, establish short-term goals for blood glucose test results, for example, 80% of readings over the next 2 weeks between 80 and 120 mg/dl, and enjoy a reward with your child if the goal is reached.

▲ When you find it necessary to call your doctor or nurse about a diabetes problem, be ready to offer one or more solutions for their consideration. This will give him or her a chance to give you feedback about your reasoning and to sharpen your skills even more.

▲ Design and conduct problem-solving experiments to see whether you and your child can identify factors that affect your child's blood glucose in predictable ways. Look at the types of foods eaten, the timing of meals, the rotation of insulin injection sites, and the amount and intensity of physical activities. Your experiment can make great science fair projects if your child is comfortable with doing that.

▲ Keep a Diabetes Problem-Solving Diary in which you record the details of any problem-solving attempts that you made. This should include a statement of the problem (for example, morning blood glucose above 220 mg/dl more than 50% of the time), an objective (80% of morning blood glucose levels below 120 mg/dl), a description of the action taken (increase evening NPH by 2 units), and the results (88% of morning blood glucose values below 120 mg/dl in the past two weeks).

▲ Actively teach adolescents with diabetes what you have learned about recognizing, defining, analyzing, and solving diabetes problems by helping them come up with solutions to situations that they, not you, have identified as problems.

▲ Solve diabetes problems *with*, rather than *for*, your teenager. When your teenager comes to you with a problem concerning blood glucose levels, ask him or her to offer a solution before you give your opinion.

New Technology: Is It Right for You?

The advances in caring for diabetes in the past two decades have been amazing, and there is every reason to believe that this trend will continue. More and more kids with type 1 diabetes are using insulin pumps for insulin delivery, new insulin types, glucose meters that can perform both blood glucose and ketone tests, and, most recently, devices that measure glucose levels almost continuously. In the near future, we will probably see more new insulin types, more accurate continuous-glucose sensors, devices that warn of looming hypoglycemia, and perhaps novel forms of insulin delivery. In the long run, I wouldn't be surprised to see an insulin pump that is regulated automatically by a continuous glucose sensor or the development of biosynthetic beta cells that can be implanted to restore insulin secretion. Perhaps there will be a day in the future when the treatment of diabetes really approaches something that could be called a cure. Along that path, every parent and every child with diabetes will probably have to ask themselves this question several times: "Is this new advance right for us and are we right for it?" Without really even knowing what specific advances are coming, I'd like to give you a general framework for helping you to make these kinds of decisions with your child and your health care team.

Here are a few suggestions that I think can make this process more successful and satisfying:

▲ Be very careful not to push your child into using any new device or method. Kids who are coerced usually don't end up cooperating very well after a few months. Be especially cautious if your child is shy about allowing his or her diabetes to become too public.

▲ Consider the effects of the new method on your child's independence and functioning away from home. Is this going to require more responsibility of your child? Is it going to make the diabetes more obvious to your child's friends? Is this going to require the school to play a more active role in your child's diabetes?

▲ Ask yourself what problems you would be trying to solve with the new method. Sometimes parents have inappropriate expectations for a technological solution to a problem that is really a behavioral or emotional issue. Also, if your current regimen is working well, remember the old adage "If it ain't broke, don't fix it."

▲ Take your time with these decisions. It's often the case that an initial product or device is followed in a few months by a better one anyway. Also, your diabetes team may be able to help you get more from a new method if they first gain a few months of direct experience using it.

▲ If you really want to try something that is brand new, ask your physician to help you enroll in a clinical research study. All new medical devices and medications are submitted to a rigorous evaluation process before they can be approved by the Food and Drug Administration for marketing.

▲ Benefit from others' experiences. Talk with and listen to health professionals who have knowledge and experience with the new methods. Hear what other parents have to say, both positive and negative. Talk to some parents who decided to go ahead with the new approach and some who decided not to and try to relate their reasons to your own situation. At the same time, realize that some people can become a little overzealous and, in their enthusiasm for some new device, medication, or approach, forget that you need to make this decision based on your situation, not theirs.

▲ Evaluate carefully whether you have the time, energy, and organization that is required to learn to use the new method, carry it out consistently and carefully, and perform troubleshooting. You need to remember that technology has the capacity both to simplify and to complicate your life. Your energy may be better spent making sure that you and your child are doing the best possible job with the tools you have right now. When you achieve that, you might find that the need for something new just seems to evaporate.

TAKE-HOME MESSAGE

7

Daily life with diabetes presents many challenges that require flexible problem-solving skills. Look at these situations as opportunities to help your child become an active diabetes problem solver, one who is able to adapt to the special problems posed by having diabetes rather than feeling resentful or overwhelmed by them.

SOCIAL SKILLS

Diabetes Problem Solving

Treatment Adherence

Managing Stress

Family Sharing of Diabetes Responsibilities

Family Communication

Emotional Coping

Diabetes Knowledge

Nick was a very overweight 15-year-old boy with type 2 diabetes. He had a hard time passing up snacks whenever they were available, but especially if he happened to be with a group of his friends. He told his mother he was afraid that if he turned down the snacks the other kids would tease him and give him a hard time about having diabetes. So he would usually have some, even though he knew eating that way would make his blood glucose too high and keep him from losing weight. With the help of their diabetes educator, Nick and his mom made up a list of all the ways his friends could help him be as healthy as possible. Nick also rehearsed some things he could say to his friends whenever they offered him food he shouldn't eat so that he could get out of some of these situations gracefully.

Nick's mom then talked to each of his closest friends and helped them see that eating snacks in front of Nick was very hard for him. Nick's mom also invited two of his friends to come with him to diabetes summer camp in a few months and they were both excited about doing that. Knowing that his friends were there to help him out gave Nick more confidence about his diabetes and helped him stick with his meal plan better than before.

8

SOCIAL SKILLS

Life with diabetes takes place in a social world populated by friends, brothers and sisters, teachers, grandparents, coaches, and strangers. When it comes to keeping diabetes in control, and adjusting to it emotionally, a lot of the action takes place away from home. Taking shots on time, testing blood glucose when necessary, dealing with low blood glucose, and making the right food choices are all responsibilities that often occur away from home. These tasks may have to compete for attention with the other social priorities of children and adolescents.

For some kids, dealing with diabetes in their social world is threatening and troublesome. They may live in fear of being seen as different, being teased because of having diabetes, having to explain diabetes to yet another new acquaintance, and facing all kinds of restrictions and limitations that their friends and classmates don't have to deal with. Other kids are confident and self-assured about their diabetes and somehow manage to encourage the important people outside of their immediate families to be helpful and supportive.

What causes children to have these very different kinds of responses to coping socially with diabetes? Getting through the emotional pain surrounding diabetes

(Key #2) is certainly important. But another important factor is the extent to which the child has the social skills necessary for dealing with peer pressure, teasing, misconceptions about diabetes, and other common dilemmas that will be encountered sooner or later by every youngster with diabetes. As with family communication, children and adolescents can be taught to improve their social skills for coping with these common roadblocks to healthy adjustment.

In this chapter, I present some of the more common social challenges that are faced by kids with diabetes and give you ideas about how youngsters can cope with these challenges. I also show you a basic strategy that will help you teach your child to develop more effective social skills, and you'll learn how to apply this approach to other social interaction trouble spots that kids might face. During this process, I define the parent's role in helping the child cultivate a network of social supports for healthy diabetes self-management.

Feeling Torn Between Diabetes and Friends

Youngsters with diabetes often find themselves in situations in which they must choose between taking good care of their diabetes, such as making healthy food choices and taking shots or doing blood glucose tests on time, versus going along with their friends and putting diabetes on the back burner. Balancing these competing priorities requires that youngsters with diabetes know how to attend gracefully to their health while being normal kids. They should remember that their true friends want them to stay healthy. At a minimum, your child's friends should know what hypoglycemia is and how to help your child if it happens. It's unfair to friends to place them in a situation where they might have to deal with a medical crisis that they don't really understand. Helping your child's friends learn more about diabetes enables them to be more supportive and helpful. Some diabetes summer camps allow campers to bring along a friend who doesn't have diabetes, which is a great vehicle for learning about diabetes.

Who to Tell About Diabetes and How

It's hard for many kids to figure out who should know about their diabetes, when they should tell them, and how to do it. This becomes a thornier problem for teenagers who have to face this issue with people they date or when they apply for jobs.

In their book, *In Control: A Guide for Teens With Diabetes*, Jean Betschart and Susan Thom give some useful suggestions for dividing people into three groups:

1. *Those who need to know:* People who need to know are those who may help your child with low blood glucose levels or who will be around when it's time for an injection. This group usually includes teachers, coaches, relatives with frequent contact, and close friends.

2. *Those who could be told:* This group is harder to define because it includes people you could tell but who don't really have to know. How do you and your child make this choice? For younger children (less than 10 years old), it's generally up to the parents to decide whom to inform about their child's diabetes and when and how to do it. How much to disclose about your child or yourself is a matter of personal preference and personality style. Without a solid reason for either informing or concealing your child's diabetes, go with the approach that makes your child more comfortable. Is the person going to learn about your child's diabetes anyway? If so, holding back may lead the person to think your child is ashamed of having diabetes. For most people in this category, it's best to wait until the topic of diabetes comes up naturally, such as when your child is questioned about eating habits or there is a need to take insulin. This is probably an easier approach than starting a conversation by telling the person about your child's diabetes.

3. *Those who don't need to know about your child's diabetes:* Those who don't need to know are people your child may see now and then but who are unlikely to be involved in things affecting your child's blood glucose level.

When Others Don't Understand Diabetes

One of the most frustrating parts of living with diabetes, for parents and children, is that you encounter people with misguided ideas about diabetes that lead them to say or do foolish things, which can be irritating and painful. This is often true about two subjects: the long-term complications of diabetes and the effects of diabetes on pregnancy. Because diabetes in its two main forms is such a common disease, many people know a friend, co-worker, or relative who has it. Sometimes people have had a limited but memorable experience with one person with diabetes that leads to lasting impressions about diabetes in general that aren't accurate. Educating others about diabetes is the key to countering these inaccuracies, but in most cases, it can only be done one person at a time. Your child needs the following tools to be equipped to deal with misconceptions about diabetes when they arise:

▲ Accurate and current diabetes knowledge

▲ Appropriate social assertiveness

▲ The realization that ignorance and hostility are not the same and that inappropriate reactions to diabetes should first be viewed as a reflection of the person's ignorance, not as an intentional insult

▲ The wisdom to know when it is necessary to challenge or correct someone's misconceptions about diabetes, which is usually needed only if that person is in a position to affect the child's future adjustment to diabetes

▲ Acceptance that most people don't need to know much about diabetes and that ignorance about diabetes will always be a part of life

Pressure to Use Alcohol, Tobacco, or Drugs

Most teens with diabetes will face the opportunity to use drugs or alcohol, smoke cigarettes, use smokeless tobacco, or engage in other risky behaviors like unprotected sex or reckless driving. There is some evidence suggesting that youngsters with diabetes, and perhaps others with chronic illnesses, may be less prone to participate in these behaviors than their peers without diabetes. Having grown up paying attention to their long-term health, choosing healthy foods, and perhaps learning some skills in how to resist peer pressure may help them avoid these problems. Kids should not be encouraged to use diabetes as an excuse, but when it comes to things like drugs, alcohol, smoking, and sex, the following statements could be made to their friends:

▲ "No thanks, my diabetes doesn't mix well with that stuff."

▲ "Hey, if you had spent as much time in your life paying attention to your health as I have, you wouldn't be doing that either."

▲ "Sorry, I can't tell if my blood glucose is low when I do that, and I don't think you guys want to spend the rest of tonight in the emergency room."

▲ "No thanks! One of my friends from diabetes camp spent a weekend in the hospital after doing that."

Few good friends will challenge a youngster with diabetes who makes a statement like one of these. Some of these statements may stretch the truth a little, but your kid's friends don't know that. With a little creativity and some suggestions from you, your youngster can rehearse comebacks like these that are effective and save face. This may be one of the few times when having diabetes can come in handy.

Dealing with Being Teased About Diabetes

Many youngsters have trouble with other kids who say or do annoying things to them just because they have diabetes. It's my experience that youngsters who tease others about having diabetes tend to have low self-esteem and feelings of inadequacy themselves, and they may often be trying to give themselves a boost by cutting down others. I try to help my young patients with diabetes recognize this, and most of them are able to point out that the teasers often harass and annoy many other kids in different ways. Don't follow any of the suggestions listed below without first learning as much as possible about the situation your child is facing and making sure that your child agrees to the approach beforehand. The solution you choose must fit your child's situation. I don't think that there is any single way of dealing with this problem that will always be effective, but here are several options to consider:

▲ Teach your child to ignore the teasing by turning away, avoiding eye contact, and perhaps speaking to someone else. This is called extinction, and it is the simplest response to describe but the hardest to carry out. It's important for you and your child to know that using this approach can result in a temporary increase in teasing as the teaser tries harder to get an emotional rise from the victim. Inconsistent use of this approach can cause teasing to get worse rather than better. But if your child can ignore teasing consistently, it will usually stop, and the teaser will move on to other, easier targets.

▲ Invite the teaser over to play after school or on a weekend, and make sure that it's during a time when your child needs to do a blood glucose test and take an insulin injection. Invite along others who don't tease about diabetes.

▲ Use modeling and role-playing to help your child practice an assertive response to the teasing. This should include teaching your child to face the teaser, maintain direct eye contact, keep a neutral and calm facial expression, speak in a firm but not angry tone of voice, and say something like "Teasing others who are different only makes you look weak, not strong, so stop."

▲ If your child is willing, get the teacher's permission for your child to do a "show and tell" for the whole class about a day in the life of a person with diabetes, or ask your diabetes educator to do it for or with your child. Once other students see that your child is not afraid or ashamed of having diabetes, the teasing often stops.

▲ Teach your child to show respect for others who are different in some way and to refuse to participate in teasing of others in any way.

▲ Make sure that your child's teacher is aware of the problem, and ask that a daily lesson be devoted to showing respect for those who differ from us.

▲ Encourage your youngster to talk to the most popular student in class and ask for that child's help in discouraging the teasing.

▲ Help your child understand that other children get teased too, only about other things.

The ABCs of Teaching Social Skills

As we grow up, we all develop our own set of habits regarding how we interact with other people. We differ in what we say, how we say it, the kinds of body language that we use, and how we start and end conversations. These are the personal characteristics that make us unique. Development of our social skills is affected a great deal by heredity, and you have probably noticed that your child has many social characteristics that remind you of yourself or the other parent.

Learning and imitation also play a big role in determining the kind of social interaction habits that children develop. Therefore, we ought to be able to use basic principles of learning and imitation to help our children develop new social skills or refine social skills that they already have. Child psychologists have been doing just that for years. Here's a basic, well-accepted framework to help you work with your child to approach other social skill problems that I haven't touched. If you're going to try this, you should start by working with your child on a relatively minor or infrequent social interaction problem, ideally one that the child recognizes as a trouble spot and hopes to correct. Also you should spend more time on the modeling and rehearsal steps when you're new at this.

▲ **Define the problem:** Describe in detail the interactions that end unpleasantly. If your child can't do this well, some options are to talk with your child's teachers or coaches about their observations or to ask your child to keep a diary about the specific social problem for a few weeks to help you learn more about it. Name the skill: It helps to give the skill a simple name that you and your child can use when talking about it. For example, if your child interrupts others a lot, you could call the targeted skill "Listening." This makes the problem an "it" rather than emphasizing that your son or daughter has a personal flaw or shortcoming, and it will make it easier for you to give feedback about the skill when you are with your child in social settings.

▲ **List the specific skill steps:** With your child's input, list the steps that the child should take when using the skill. Write down examples of a script of what the child should say when using this skill, and make sure that your child understands the reason for each part of the script.

▲ **Describe the nonverbal parts of the skill:** With your child's input, write down a list of the basic "body language" parts of the skill. For all social skills, this should include facing the other person, making and keeping eye contact with the other person, and keeping a straight body posture. It's also a good idea for the list to include a description of facial expression and tone of voice.

▲ **List cues for using the skill:** Help your child make a list of the social situations in which the skill should be used. Try to define the characteristics of that situation in such a way that your child will know if it's time to use the skill. Also, help your child anticipate any situations in which using the skill would be inappropriate.

▲ **Model the skill for your child:** Show your child exactly what it looks like and sounds like when the skill is used properly and improperly. Model good and bad examples of the skill and ask your child to evaluate each example.

▲ **Have your child rehearse the skill:** Role-play typical situations in which the skill should be used, and give your child feedback about his or her demonstration of the skill. Practice many examples of different situations until you are satisfied that your child knows how to use the skill correctly.

▲ **Reinforce using the skill:** Have your child self-monitor the effectiveness of the skill when it was used. Role-play with your child any situations in which the skill wasn't used as planned or didn't have the intended effect. Don't make changes to any of the skill components until you first make sure that your child is still using the skill as it was originally learned.

▲ **Praise your child for trying to work on this difficult problem:** It really helps a lot of kids just to know that their parents are supportive and involved and that there are options open to them that they hadn't yet considered or tried.

TAKE-HOME MESSAGE

8 Children with diabetes need skills for dealing with common social challenges that they may face and for developing a helpful and supportive social network. You can help your child to learn better social skills.

SCHOOL ADJUSTMENT

Social Skills

Diabetes Problem Solving

Treatment Adherence

Managing Stress

Family Sharing of Diabetes Responsibilities

Family Communication

Emotional Coping

Diabetes Knowledge

Jasmine was diagnosed with type 1 diabetes when she was only about 2 years old and it was very difficult to keep her diabetes in good control for the first 2 to 3 years. Early in her 3rd grade school year, her teacher referred her for an evaluation because her reading skills were not up to grade level. The school psychologist found that Jasmine had missed learning some important skills, most importantly the skills to process basic sounds that make up our language and the ability to understand the sounds associated with letters of the alphabet and with pairs of letters. She was given special tutoring throughout that school year to help her re-learn those basic skills. By the end of the school year, she had caught up and was reading at grade level.

SCHOOL ADJUSTMENT

School is an important influence for all children. School-aged children spend about 1,100 hours per year at school, and possibly many more depending on their involvement in sports or other organized activities. Diabetes doesn't go away during those times, and having diabetes can complicate the life of a student in many ways. Statistically speaking, each elementary school teacher is likely to have a student with diabetes about once in every twenty years of teaching. Consequently, educators are not necessarily well prepared for the special issues that are raised by children with chronic illnesses such as diabetes.

As discussed in the previous chapter, there are many special social situations that your child may face in school. Some children may have difficulty with returning to school after first being diagnosed. Teachers, coaches, and other students with limited knowledge about diabetes can carry around misconceptions about the disease that lead to inappropriate treatment of children with diabetes. Some students may tease the child about having diabetes.

In addition to these social challenges, youngsters with diabetes may be faced with other potential hurdles. Children with any chronic disease are more likely to be absent from school because of both actual symptoms of the disease and frequent medical appointments. About 7% of elementary school students have learning disorders, and so do at least that many children with diabetes. For a variety of reasons, the combination of diabetes and learning disorders can pose some thorny problems and be a source of worry and confusion to families and teachers. Concerns about safety can lead to well-meaning but overprotective and unnecessarily restrictive practices. School personnel may be guilty of "diabetism" by interpreting the child's characteristics, such as emotionality, disorganization, or inattention, as manifestations of diabetes rather than simply a feature of the child's personality. Occasionally, children with diabetes develop a pattern (sometimes called *school phobia*) in which the child avoids school attendance, consciously or not, through poor diabetic control.

Parents and teachers face some pretty big challenges in preventing, recognizing, and correcting these situations. In this chapter, I discuss each of these school concerns in more detail and provide some practical suggestions that may help parents work with teachers and other school personnel to meet these challenges for their children.

Please keep in mind the points and practical suggestions made in the previous chapter regarding the need for children with diabetes to develop social skills that can help them cope with the typical social challenges that accompany life with diabetes. Although many of those points pertain primarily to your child's adjustment to school, they are not repeated here.

Educating Classmates and Teachers About Diabetes

If your youngster is newly diagnosed with diabetes, you can do him or her a big favor by helping the child's teacher and classmates learn a little about diabetes. There really isn't that much that school staff need to know medically about diabetes beyond learning how to recognize and help out during a low blood glucose reaction and maybe how a blood glucose test is done. But there are some other points that should be made as early as possible:

▲ Diabetes is not contagious or preventable.

▲ Your child will still be able to live like a normal kid in almost every way.

▲ Your child should be treated just like before the diabetes was diagnosed.

Make the process of educating teachers and classmates an annual task. I suggest that you and your child together draw from the following options as ways of promoting your child's safety in school and adaptation to diabetes while there. Schedule a meeting with your child's teachers, and perhaps the school nurse or health aide, before each school year begins. Provide a letter from your child's physician, as well as pamphlets and other educational materials on what the teacher needs to know about diabetes. For younger children, parents can offer to do a classroom talk or demonstration on living with diabetes or enlist a member of the diabetes team to do so. There are also suitable videotapes that could be used for this purpose (see the "Resources" section).

When possible, suggest that your child use diabetes as the topic for assignments such as speeches, term papers, and science projects. Recruit members of your diabetes team to speak at school career days or to address your child's class about diabetes. Take advantage of recreational opportunities for children with diabetes that allow them to bring along a friend who does not have diabetes. In addition to summer camps, many diabetes organizations hold parties, field trips, or fund-raising events that provide these kinds of opportunities.

Dealing with Diabetism

You're probably familiar with racism and sexism. These are two social institutions that share some common features. Both are characterized by the belief or attitude that a single characteristic defines an individual's identity so completely that it determines everything the person does, thinks, or feels. Both end up unnecessarily restricting the range of opportunities and experiences not only of the "victim," but also of the person who holds the attitude.

People with diabetes have to contend with a similar process that I call *diabetism*, the tendency to define a person with diabetes first as a "diabetic" and second as a person. This certainly doesn't happen only at school, but that's where I've run into many examples of it. I don't know how common diabetism is, but I think that it can be just as incapacitating and frustrating to children with diabetes as racism or sexism can be to other children. Here are some examples of diabetism:

▲ A high school basketball player is benched when his new coach learns that he has diabetes.

▲ A teacher criticizes a student with diabetes in class by saying, "Pay attention! What's the matter—is your blood glucose too low?"

▲ A school counselor advises an above-average student with diabetes against pursuing a college prep curriculum.

▲ Classmates of a 13-year-old girl with diabetes remark that her recent irritability and emotional fluctuations must be due to her diabetes.

▲ A student with diabetes is not allowed to be a member of the school safety patrol.

▲ A student's mother discourages her daughter from playing after school with "that diabetic girl."

Usually, instances of diabetism are due to a lack of awareness and knowledge of diabetes, and if the issue is raised calmly and objectively, the person responsible more often than not apologizes and changes his or her behavior in the future. If diabetist behavior by a school staff member persists after your initial discussion about it, I recommend pursuing it further with the school principal or other administrative official.

Learning Disabilities and Diabetes

Many parents want to know if there is any connection between diabetes and learning disorders or school performance. This question is a lot more complicated than it sounds. The term *learning disability* refers to a disorder of learning or expression of basic academic skills such as arithmetic, reading, or spoken or written language. It is defined most often as a significant discrepancy between a child's learning potential (IQ) and academic progress (as measured by standardized achievement tests) that cannot be attributed to other factors such as vision or hearing impairment, language or cultural barriers, or poor school attendance. In most states, a child's academic achievement must be two or more grade levels below their current grade placement to be identified as learning disabled. About 7% of all school-aged children will be categorized as learning disabled at some time during their school years, so it is quite common. The vast majority of learning-disabled people become productive, independently functioning adults who lead full and satisfying lives. Although many people with learning disabilities may have lifelong difficulty with specific academic skills, most find ways to compensate for these problems, such as pursuing employment in positions that do not require extensive use of that skill. There are many famous people who had learning disabilities but who managed to make outstanding contributions to their respective fields.

In the past decade, there have been several research studies showing that children who are diagnosed with diabetes when younger than seven may be at an increased risk of having learning disabilities later in life. There also appears to be a higher risk of learning disabilities among boys with diabetes than among girls. Although the research has been fairly consistent in finding some evidence of learning problems in these select groups of children with diabetes, the specific nature of the learning problems that were found has differed in different studies. None of the studies has determined exactly why the risk of learning disabilities increases in these children. Researchers have asked whether this association occurs because of some aspect of diabetes, such as severe hypoglycemia, episodes of diabetic ketoacidosis, prolonged high blood glucose, or simply duration of diabetes, or whether early onset of diabetes and learning disabilities may simply be traits that are inherited together. Because many of these factors are highly correlated with one another, it's been difficult for researchers to determine the possible contributions of each factor separately. Until these questions can be answered, many doctors are trying to *minimize* the frequency of severe hypoglycemia among very young children with diabetes because that is widely considered to be the culprit. Studies of this question have yielded somewhat conflicting results and there is evidence both that severe hypoglycemia is and is not associated with the later emergence of learning difficulties in children with diabetes.

Regardless of whether diabetes somehow causes or unmasks learning disabilities, and what the precise cause is, it is very important to recognize these problems as early as possible and to take steps to correct or compensate for them. Children diagnosed with either learning disabilities or attention problems may have extra trouble with handling their diabetes treatment and monitoring responsibilities consistently. Disorders of learning and attention affect basic concentration, memory, organizational skills, and the ability to control impulses, all of which can interfere with effective diabetes self-management. Self-care responsibilities for youngsters with these types of problems may need to be reduced in accord with the severity of their difficulties, and parents should take care to ensure that the child is completing self-care tasks accurately and consistently.

Effective medical and psychological treatments are widely available for children diagnosed with attention deficit hyperactivity disorder (ADHD), a syndrome characterized by high levels of inattention, hyperactivity, and poor impulse control. There is no evidence that ADHD is any more *common* among children with diabetes, but it is prevalent among children in general. Children with diabetes who also have ADHD may have more success in diabetes self-care if these complicating problems are addressed and controlled. This is usually possible with some combination of family counseling, behavior modification, appropriate school placement, and medication. The most commonly used medications for children with ADHD (Ritalin, Dexedrine, Adderal, and Cylert) are all stimulants that can increase blood glucose levels by causing the liver and kidneys to release stored glucose. However, this minor effect can usually be offset easily by insulin dosage adjustments, so there is little reason to deprive a child with ADHD and diabetes of medication treatment if there is good evidence he or she would benefit from them.

School Avoidance

A small percentage of school-age children show a cluster of symptoms that are commonly called "school phobia" or "school avoidance," which refers to repeated absence from school coupled with intense anxiety or aversion toward school attendance. It is often accompanied by vague or fleeting physical symptoms, such as headaches and abdominal pain, and these complaints are often the main cause of the absences. Children with diabetes are not immune to school avoidance, and when these symptoms are combined with poorly controlled diabetes, the result can be repeated hospitalizations, an expensive pursuit of medical causes, and deterioration of the trust between the health care team, the school, and the family. Recognizing and/or preventing school avoidance in the child with diabetes is therefore an important responsibility shared by the parents, the health care team, and the school.

This school avoidance syndrome has some fairly consistent features. The child usually has a history of repeated school absences, often following a vague physical ailment. There is often rapid improvement in the physical symptoms after removing the child from school. The pattern of physical symptoms typically occurs much less frequently, if at all, when school is not in session. Extensive medical evaluation usually yields no clear physical explanation. The child appears to enjoy medical attention and hospitalizations or is indifferent to the severity of the health problems. Interestingly, school-avoidant children often have above-average grades and a stated desire to attend school. There is often evidence of past or current anxiety about separating from parents. I do not assume that the child who is resisting school attendance is doing so on purpose or that the physical symptoms aren't real. In fact, many of these children, particularly those who are less mature socially or who do not have strong coping skills, may be reacting physically to intense anxiety associated with school performance, social acceptance, or both.

With these points in mind, if your child with diabetes appears to have most of the above characteristics you should be prepared to carry out a multi-pronged approach to help your child adjust to regular school attendance and participation. You must insist on daily school attendance unless an adult can verify a physical symptom, such as vomiting, diarrhea, or fever. Provide daily positive reinforcement for your child's school attendance in the form of extra privileges or treats. Minimize your child's opportunities for entertaining, fun, or stimulating activities on days of school absence. Avoid so-called homebound instruction, in which a teacher visits your child at home a few times per week to keep up with schoolwork. It is often extremely difficult to return school-avoidant children to regular school attendance once they have experienced this type of situation. Obtain a letter from your child's physician to the school, stipulating clearly the precise conditions under which you should be called to bring the child home. Consider evaluation by a mental health professional regarding possible causes of your child's anxiety related to school and the possible need for individual therapy. Ask your school to develop an Accommodation Plan under Section 504 of the Rehabilitation Act of 1973 that puts the above steps into a formal, legally binding agreement.

Special Education and Other Alternatives

Federal laws and regulations governing special education require school systems that receive federal funds to make reasonable accommodations for the special needs of its students. But getting this done in a timely and consistent manner sometimes isn't so easy. Public schools must offer appropriate special education placements to students who have any of eight handicapping conditions, including:

▲ Learning disabilities

▲ Mental retardation

▲ Severe behavior disorders

▲ Autism

▲ Visual impairment

▲ Hearing impairment

▲ Orthopedic disabilities

▲ Health impairment

This last category can include a chronic physical illness such as diabetes if it can be shown to impede the child's ability to learn in a normal classroom setting. However, special education programs may not offer a sufficiently challenging curriculum to satisfy many parents. For children who do not meet eligibility requirements for special education programs, another alternative that can be helpful is Section 504 of the Rehabilitation Act. Children with certain handicapping conditions, of which diabetes is an example, are eligible for written, individualized "accommodation plans," which require the school to make reasonable changes in the child's schedule, curriculum, or classroom routines, that are necessary to accommodate to the child's handicap and that promote the child's ability to be educated. Accommodation plans have been used to enable children with diabetes to perform blood glucose tests when needed, eat snacks as scheduled, and have supplies for treating hypoglycemia available in school. If your child's diabetes management has been a barrier to his or her education in some way, ask your school principal to put you in touch with the person who is responsible for monitoring your school district's compliance with the Section 504 requirements.

Homeschooling: Why and Why Not

There is also a rapidly growing national trend for parents to function as their own children's teachers at home. Although laws and regulations vary in different states, parents can take advantage of this alternative if they want to and are willing to abide by approved procedures. At one time, only certified teachers could "home-school" their children, although this is generally no longer the case. Some parents of children with chronic illnesses find this to be a good alternative to the hassles encountered in trying to adapt the typical classroom setting to the special needs of these children.

In homeschooling, one of the child's parents or other adult caregiver is approved by the public school system to function as the child's teacher. Ordinarily, this requires the use of a specified curriculum and periodic achievement testing to ensure that the child is making acceptable academic progress. I never recommend homeschooling solely because a child has diabetes, but this is a decision that requires careful family consideration. Although I don't advocate homeschooling across the board, it can be a reasonable alternative for families to consider if these circumstances exist:

▲ The parent who will do the teaching understands that he or she is making a long-term commitment to several hours of daily instruction of their child.

▲ Your child shows no signs of a learning disability.

▲ Your child participates actively in several other structured sources of healthy social interactions with peers in activities such as sports, hobbies, church youth groups, or scouting programs.

▲ Your child shows absolutely no symptoms of school avoidance as defined earlier in this chapter.

▲ The parent-teacher has sufficient skills to teach the required curriculum to the child and a calm and tolerant temperament that enables teaching the child with a minimum of frustration or tension.

If all of these things are in place, homeschooling can be immensely successful and productive. In fact, some research shows that homeschooled children perform better on standardized tests of academic achievement than do those who attended regular schools. At the same time, there are some bad reasons to make the decision to homeschool your child:

▲ Your child doesn't get along with other children at the school.

▲ Your child's teacher has shown insufficient attention to your child's special needs regarding diabetes care in the school.

▲ You have had conflict with teachers or administrators at your child's school.

These "bad" reasons share one common feature. They are motivated negatively by avoidance of a real or perceived problem. I believe that the decision to homeschool your child should be based only on positive and constructive reasons. Teaching your child to leave problematic situations because they are difficult or frustrating may be sending a message that you don't really intend to send. Wouldn't it be a healthier lesson for your child to demonstrate how problems with others can be fixed if we just try hard enough?

TAKE-HOME MESSAGE

9

Children with diabetes face several special challenges in school. You should recognize these challenges, be an advocate for your child in school, and teach your child how to be appropriately assertive regarding his or her unique needs in school.

KEY
10

RELATING
TO HEALTH
PROFESSIONALS

School Adjustment

Social Skills

Diabetes Problem Solving

Treatment Adherence

Managing Stress

Family Sharing of Diabetes Responsibilities

Family Communication

Emotional Coping

Diabetes Knowledge

Jeff was a 21-year-old college student who was diagnosed with diabetes at age seven. His schedule at college is very inconsistent and he had a lot of trouble figuring out how to fit his diabetes self-care into his hectic life.

Because he hadn't seen a doctor regularly for his diabetes since starting college, Jeff was on his own when it came to making sense of his blood glucose levels and adjusting his insulin dose to his activity and eating habits. He had an episode of severe hypoglycemia that landed him in the emergency room and required an overnight hospital stay. During that hospitalization, his doctor set him up with follow-up appointments with the diabetes team at the university's medical school.

Since establishing a more consistent relationship with a health care team, Jeff was started on a more flexible regimen consisting of one daily injection of glargine (Lantus) at bedtime and injections of short-acting insulin before meals based on his blood sugar level and the amount of carbohydrate he planned to eat. His diabetic control has been excellent ever since.

RELATING TO HEALTH PROFESSIONALS

Every person with diabetes faces a lifetime of relating to health care professionals. Because the quality of those relationships affects both physical and mental health outcomes, it is important that children and adolescents with diabetes learn effective ways of interacting with health care professionals. Few families make an obvious, intentional effort to teach their children with diabetes how to relate to doctors and nurses, but it's important for parents to realize that every time you interact with a member of the health care team, you are teaching your child by your example. In this chapter, I provide several specific examples of ways in which parents can use health care interactions as a vehicle for teaching their children how to establish trusting, honest, and satisfying relationships with health care professionals.

Teaching Your Child to Be an Active Health Care Consumer

Many people interact differently with health care professionals, especially their physicians, compared to how they interact with attorneys, accountants, homebuilders, plumbers, or other service providers. Most people probably wouldn't let these other professionals monopolize a conversation. Most would probably be quick to interrupt if the professional used a technical term that they didn't understand. Most people would make sure that all of their questions were answered before they agreed to receive a professional's services. But when talking to doctors, many people are less communicative, more prone to accept statements without question, and less likely to interrupt. They may leave the clinic visit feeling that the physician did not give sufficient time to address their main concerns.

But things are changing, especially for young people with chronic illnesses like diabetes. Modern training of doctors and other health professionals emphasizes the importance of good communication and the effectiveness of treating these illnesses with a team of health professionals from different fields. More and more research has shown that the quality of physician-patient interaction and communication affects patients' adherence to treatment and health outcomes, and doctors, as well as other health professionals, are paying attention.

Young people with diabetes need to develop skills as health care consumers to maximize their ability to stay in good health for a lifetime. The main influence on how effectively your child will develop these skills is how you behave during clinic visits and telephone conversations with health professionals. Ask yourself these questions:

▲ Are you an active and assertive health care consumer?

▲ Do you come to clinic visits prepared with problems and questions to be addressed during the visit?

▲ During clinic visits and telephone calls, is communication from you just about as frequent as communication to you?

▲ During clinic visits, do you ask specific questions to the health professionals?

▲ Do you feel there is a good match between the personalities and styles of members of the health care team with your own needs and style?

▲ Are you able to describe diabetes and its treatment accurately and understand the role of each part of the treatment plan?

▲ Do you state honestly and directly if there is an aspect of the treatment plan that is unclear, unacceptable, or impossible?

▲ Do you make it clear when the goals of treatment expressed by the health care team differ from yours in any way?

To many of you, these ideas may seem like quite a change from the kind of health care that you're used to. And not all health care professionals are comfortable with patients who are assertive and active health care consumers. Those who are, however, describe their relationships with their patients as more trusting, more thera-peutic, more personal, and less stressful.

It's never too early to begin teaching your child how to become an active, independent health care consumer. Even very young chil-dren have a role to play by cooperating with examination proce-dures during health care encounters and by trying to help the health care provider to understand their symptoms. School-age children can learn to report on their symptoms and diabetes management when they are in school or otherwise away from home, and they can begin to develop the confidence necessary to carry on conversations with health professionals. Teenagers can assert their independence by answering questions about their diabetes, by requesting to be seen by the physician without their parents present, and by learning to make telephone calls to members of the diabetes team. Let's con-sider your role as a parent in encouraging your child with diabetes to develop these skills.

Teaching by Example

The best method for teaching your child with diabetes to become an active health care consumer is to be one yourself. Here are some specific things for you to do to provide this kind of example for your children with diabetes:

▲ Keep a notebook at home for recording issues that need to be dis-cussed with members of your health care team at your next clinic visit or by telephone. Take the notebook to clinic visits, and write down the answers to your questions.

▲ Be honest and direct in conversations with members of your health care team.

▲ At the end of clinic visits, repeat the key information that you thought you heard to enable the health care professional to reinforce or correct your recollection.

▲ After the clinic visit, discuss with your child what occurred, and give the opportunity for questions.

Transferring Responsibility for Health Care to Your Teenager

At some point in middle adolescence, your teenager with diabetes will be ready to begin assuming responsibility for tasks such as making and keeping clinic appointments, deciding when to call a health professional, and getting prescriptions filled. Many parents wait too long to start this process and then are forced to rush through teaching their youngsters how to do these things. The gradual process of transferring responsibility can begin early, perhaps around age 11 or 12 years for some children. Below, I've laid out a reasonable sequence of steps in the process of transferring the responsibility for interacting with health care professionals from parents to adolescents in a way that is safe, effective, and likely to promote your child's self-confidence.

▲ Sometime during late childhood or early adolescence, begin asking your child to write down specific issues or questions that should be discussed at the next clinic visit. At about this time, allow your child to participate in telephone conversations that you might have with a member of the health care team.

▲ In early adolescence (about 11 or 12 years of age), begin asking your child to answer some of the more basic questions asked by health professionals during clinic visits. The older your adolescent becomes, the less willing you should be to solve problems for him or her. When problems appear, your first reaction should be to ask your teenager to come up with several ways in which the problem might be solved, to evaluate each projected solution, and to justify the chosen solution.

▲ In mid-adolescence (about 14 or 15 years of age), begin asking your child to answer most of the questions posed by members of the health care team during clinic visits.

▲ When your child reaches late adolescence (about age 16), ask your health care team to spend at least part of each clinic visit alone with your child. Gradually increase this amount of time over the next one to two years.

▲ Once your child has obtained a driver's license, it's time to expect the child to make clinic appointments with your supervision and assistance.

▲ During late adolescence, your child should be given permission to make necessary telephone calls to members of the health care team.

Graduating to Adult Health Care

In general, most healthy people in their late teens and early 20s don't find themselves in doctor's offices very frequently. Health care use in this age-group tends to be unplanned, intermittent, and crisis-oriented, with little continuity from visit to visit as to the health care provider used or the location of health care delivery. Studies of health care-use patterns among late adolescents with diabetes reveal some pretty alarming trends and indicate that things really aren't much different for them, despite the fact that they have a lifelong chronic illness. Around the time that teenagers get their drivers' licenses, the frequency of visits to the diabetes clinic begins to decline. This often seems to continue well into their early 20s.

My colleagues and I studied a group of 81 young adults who had "graduated" from a multidisciplinary pediatric diabetes program and had gone on to adult health care. To summarize our results from that study, those young adults who had bad experiences controlling their diabetes during earlier adolescence, perhaps chronically poor treatment adherence with multiple hospitalizations, tended to show the most sporadic health care use during early adulthood. Typically, these young adults received occasional health care services from a variety of sources and didn't stick with any specific clinic or team for a substantial period. Therefore, those who were probably most in need of a well-planned and coordinated transition to adult health care were the least likely to experience it.

Many teenagers with diabetes may prefer to remain under the care of their familiar pediatricians and diabetes teams. Others may want to move on to adult health care settings, and in some instances, this may be required by insurance policies or clinic procedures. If your son or daughter falls into one of these categories, there are several things that you can do to increase the chances that he or she will continue to make effective use of available health care services into early adulthood.

By the time your child is 16 years old, start working with your current physician to plan a transfer to a physician who specializes in treating adults with diabetes. Involve your teenager from the start in the process of selecting a personal physician and health care team. Encourage your teenager, starting in early adolescence, to identify features of clinics, treatment practices, or personal characteristics of health professionals that are most important in selecting a new physician or team. Tell your doctor and other members of your diabetes team about your child's preferences, and ask them to suggest health care professionals for your child and you to consider. As an alternative, ask your local American Diabetes Association affiliate for a list of physicians and diabetes clinics in your area.

If possible, help your teenager make an appointment for a pre-transfer visit with the top one or two physicians or teams on your list to finalize your decision. If the physician or clinic won't agree to this, look elsewhere. Ask your doctor to write a formal letter of referral to the physician that you decide on, and include the letter with other health records.

Preconception Counseling

A conservative estimate is that about 75% to 80% of teenaged girls in the United States are sexually active by the time they graduate from high school. This information is even more disturbing in the light of reports that adolescents' knowledge of pregnancy, contraception, and reproductive health is generally poor. The few studies of these issues among young women with diabetes suggest that the same general conclusions probably apply to them. Tremendous progress has been made in the past 20 years that has helped increase the chances of successful pregnancies and healthy babies for young women with diabetes. But the fact remains that achieving these happy outcomes requires excellent glucose control before and at the time of conception and that this excellent control be maintained throughout the pregnancy. Poor diabetic control at conception increases the risk that the baby will be born with serious, possibly fatal, health problems. Consequently, each pregnancy of a woman with diabetes should be planned, and every planned pregnancy should be preceded by an intense team effort to establish and maintain near-normal blood glucose levels.

The importance of preconception counseling for young women with diabetes cannot be overemphasized. Parents of girls with diabetes may need to be advocates for their daughters to ensure either that this service is provided or that a referral is made to someone who is qualified to do so. I suspect that too often preconception counseling is not offered to girls with diabetes until after they have become sexually active. Education about the need for excellent blood glucose levels before and during pregnancy should begin in early to middle adolescence.

Locating a Qualified Mental Health Professional

If you need to obtain the services of a qualified mental health professional, it's important that you know how to locate one who can help your family cope with diabetes. There are many different kinds of professionals who can provide these kinds of services, so sometimes it can get a little confusing when parents try to find the person who matches their child's needs. Here is a description of several common mental health professions. In "Resources," I have listed some organizations that can provide referrals to mental health professionals near you.

▲ **Psychologists** hold a PhD degree in psychology that requires four to five years of graduate school after obtaining a Bachelor's degree. Psychologists must have one or two years of supervised clinical experience to qualify for a license and this requirement varies among the states. Psychologists may not prescribe medications and usually cannot admit patients to psychiatric hospitals, although some exceptions to these rules are emerging. Many psychologists have specialized training and experience in clinical child psychology and restrict their practices to children and adolescents. Others, often referred to as pediatric psychologists, work in children's medical care settings.

▲ **Psychiatrists** are licensed physicians who have completed 4 years of medical school followed by at least 3 years of residency training in psychiatry. They are able to prescribe medications and admit patients to psychiatric hospitals. Some psychiatrists pursue additional training to obtain board certification as a Child and Adolescent Psychiatrist.

▲ **Social Workers** must hold a Master's Degree in Social Work, requiring 2 to 3 years of postgraduate study, to be licensed to offer clinical services. Many social workers who hold certification as a LCSW (Licensed Clinical Social Worker) or LISW (Licensed Independent Social Worker) are able to engage in independent clinical practice.

▲ **Behavioral-Developmental Pediatricians** are board-certified pediatricians who have completed medical school and a 3-year residency in pediatrics and who have gone on to another 3 years of training in children's behavioral and developmental disorders. They are often affiliated with departments of pediatrics in medical schools or large children's hospitals.

▲ **Psychiatric Nurses** have completed nursing school and obtained a license as a Registered Nurse and then pursued additional training in psychiatric nursing.

▲ **Counselors and Psychotherapists** may hold a variety of masters or doctoral degrees in such fields as counseling, educational psychology, social work, vocational rehabilitation, and related professions. Most states provide a mechanism allowing properly trained and experienced professionals with these other kinds of training to offer clinical services within their areas of expertise.

Your health insurance plan may place restrictions on which providers of mental health services may be covered under your policy. If you have the luxury of choosing the mental health professional whom you will work with, here are some steps to finding the best-qualified person whose training and experience suits your needs:

▲ Ask a member of your child's diabetes health care team for a referral to a mental health professional. Alternatively, ask other parents of youngsters with diabetes about their experiences in your area.

▲ It's ideal if you can find someone who has experience working with youngsters with diabetes or other chronic childhood diseases like asthma, cancer, or epilepsy. If no specific person has established a close working relationship with your diabetes health care team, it may take more effort on your part to find a qualified professional. Because adult diabetes is more common, it may be possible to find a qualified professional who has worked with adult patients with diabetes. Your local American Diabetes Association affiliate may be able to steer you in the right direction.

▲ If you can't find someone with those kinds of training or experience, you should try to find a mental health professional who has skills in child behavior therapy, cognitive behavior therapy, and/or family therapy techniques. These are the methods that have been most clearly confirmed as effective for the typical kinds of problems that are shown by children and adolescents with diabetes.

▲ If none of these avenues works for you, contact one of the national organizations listed in the Resources section for a list of qualified professionals in your region. If the mental health professional that you select has no experience with childhood diabetes, loaning him or her this book might be a good starting point. There are also many references in the Resources section that may be of interest.

TAKE-HOME MESSAGE

10

Because every child with diabetes faces a lifetime of relationships with health professionals, your child needs to learn how to develop a good working partnership with a health care team. Every health care interaction is a chance for you to teach your child these important skills.

PUTTING IT ALL TOGETHER

I have laid out 10 important tasks for healthy adjustment to diabetes, from the most fundamental to the more specialized, that are posed to families by virtue of raising a child with diabetes. I'm sure that many, if not most, of you who read this book are thinking that living with diabetes is far more complicated than it sounded at first. That's certainly my reaction after working with so many families for the past 23 years! Don't let the complexity of the challenge discourage you. Most families adapt to these tasks fairly well the first time around and don't find themselves fighting the same battles over and over again. Many of you have probably already skated through some of the tasks without even realizing what an awesome responsibility you had and what a complex challenge you were facing.

With this book I've given you dozens of practical suggestions. I know they are practical because I've seen most of them work for many families. None of them are universally effective, but if you keep trying, you can often adapt or combine some of these suggestions into something that works for you and your family. The fact is that most of the challenges discussed in this book don't go away if they are ignored, but they do tend to improve if working on them together remains a family priority. If things don't work out for you and your family in trying to tackle one or more of these tasks, I hope that this book has helped to acquaint you with how a mental health professional might be able to help. Many people feel awkward about seeking mental health services, but doing your best as a parent means getting a little help. We get driver's education before getting a driver's license. Plumbers, dog groomers, electricians, and real estate agents all must have training and pass exams before they are licensed to practice their trades. What is it about parenting that we think it should come naturally to all adults?

Raising a child with diabetes is a balancing act that challenges families with 10 tasks that are fundamental to healthy physical and psychological adjustment to diabetes. Maintaining accurate knowledge about diabetes, coping with the emotional pain of having the disease, effectively managing other stresses that get in the way of good self-care, and productive family communication form the foundation for the other tasks. Coping successfully with these tasks makes the remaining tasks that much easier, whereas failing to do so makes the other tasks difficult. Families who cope successfully with diabetes and who raise a physically and mentally healthy youngster with diabetes tend to do so by drawing flexibly from a wide variety of coping skills and styles. I hope that this book provides you with the knowledge and practical ideas you need to be the best possible parent for your child with diabetes.

Where do you go from here? After you read this book refer to it regularly to help you keep things on track. Take it off the shelf every now and then, at least once a year, and leaf through the 10 Take Home Messages. I also encourage you to loan it to your child's teachers, grandparents, coaches, or any other adult who could play an important role in helping your child make the most of life with diabetes.

RESOURCES

Additional Reading

Listed below are some additional resources for those interested in more detailed discussion of the issues raised in each chapter. Some of these references are to original research articles, whereas others are review articles or book chapters. The easiest way to obtain these references is through a university or medical center library. Few of them will be readily available at public libraries.

Journals

Key #1: Diabetes Knowledge

Johnson SB: Insulin-dependent diabetes mellitus in childhood. In M. C. Roberts (Ed.), *Handbook of Pediatric Psychology* (pp. 263–285). New York, Guilford Press, 1995

Johnson SB, Pollak T, Silverstein JH, Rosenbloom A, Spillar R, McCallum M, Harkavy J: Cognitive and behavioral knowledge about insulin-dependent diabetes mellitus among children and their parents. *Pediatrics* 69:708–24, 1982

Key #2: Emotional Coping

Kovacs M, Goldston D, Obrosky DS, Bonar LK: Psychiatric disorders in youths with IDDM: rates and risk factors. *Diabetes Care* 20:36–44, 1997

Kovacs M, Lyengar S, Goldston D, Obrosky DS, Stewart J, Marsh J: Psychological functioning among mothers of children with insulin-dependent diabetes mellitus. *Journal of Consulting and Clinical Psychology* 58:159–65, 1990

Wysocki T, Huxtable KS, Linscheid TR, Wayne W: Adjustment to diabetes mellitus in preschoolers and their mothers. *Diabetes Care* 12:524–29, 1989

Key #3: Family Communication

Bobrow ES, AvRuskin TW, Siller J: Mother-daughter interaction and adherence to diabetes regimens. *Diabetes Care* 8:146–51, 1985

Robin AL, Foster SL: *Negotiating Parent-Adolescent Conflict: A Behavioral-Family Systems Approach.* New York, Guilford, 1989

Wysocki T: Associations among parent-adolescent relationships, metabolic control and adjustment to diabetes in adolescents. *Journal of Pediatric Psychology* 18:443–54, 1993

Key #4: Family Sharing of Diabetes Responsibilities

Anderson BJ, Auslaiider WF, Jung KC, Miller JP, Santiago JV: Assessing family sharing of diabetes responsibilities. *Journal of Pediatric Psychology 1* 5:477–92, 1990

Anderson BJ, Brackett J, Ho J, Laffel L: An office-based intervention to maintain parent-adolescent teamwork in diabetes management: impact on parent involvement, family conflict, and subsequent glycemic control. *Diabetes Care* 22:713–21, 1999

Follansbee DM: Assuming responsibility for diabetes management: What age? What price? *The Diabetes Educator* 15:347–52, 1989

La Greca AM, Follansbee DM, Skyler JS: Developmental and behavioral aspects of diabetes management in youngsters. *Children's Health Care* 19:132–39, 1990

Wysocki T, Taylor A, Hough BS, Linscheid TR, Yeates KO, Naglieri, JA: Deviation from developmentally appropriate self-care autonomy: association with diabetes outcomes. *Diabetes Care* 19:119–25, 1996

Key #5: Managing Stress

Delamater AM, Kurtz SC, Bubb J, White NH, Santiago JV: Stress and coping in relation to metabolic control of adolescents with type 1 diabetes mellitus. *Journal of Developmental and Behavioral Pediatrics* 8:136–40, 1987

Hanson CL, Henggeler SW, Burghen G: Social competence and parental support as mediators of the link between stress and metabolic control in adolescents with insulin-dependent diabetes mellitus. *Journal of Consulting and Clinical Psychology* 55:529–33, 1987

White K, Kolman ML, Wexler P, Polin G, Winter Rj: Unstable diabetes and unstable families: a psychosocial evaluation of children with recurrent diabetic ketoacidosis. *Pediatrics* 73:749–55, 1984

Key #6: Treatment Adherence

Diabetes Control and Complications Trial Research Group: Effect of intensive diabetes treatment on the development and progression of long-term complications in adolescents with insulin-dependent diabetes mellitus: Diabetes Control and Complications Trial. *Journal of Pediatrics* 125:177–88, 1994

Jacobson AM, Hauser ST, Lavori P, Wolfsdorf JI, Herskowitz RD, Milley JE, Bliss R, Gelfand E, Wertlieb D, Stein J: Adherence among children and adolescents with insulin-dependent diabetes mellitus over a four-year longitudinal follow-up: the influence of patient coping and adjustment. *Journal of Pediatric Psychology* 15:511–26, 1990

Johnson SB: Insulin-dependent diabetes mellitus in childhood. In M. C. Roberts (Ed.), *Handbook of Pediatric Psychology* (pp. 263–285). New York, Guilford Press, 1995

Weissberg-Benchell J, Glasgow AM, Tynan WD, Wirtz P, Turek J, Ward J: Adolescent diabetes management and mismanagement. *Diabetes Care* 18:77–82, 1995

Wysocki T, Green LB, Huxtable KS: Blood glucose monitoring by diabetic adolescents: compliance and metabolic control. *Health Psychology* 8:267–84, 1989

Key #7: Diabetes Problem Solving

Anderson BJ, Wolf FM, Burkhart MT, Cornell RG, Bacon GE: Effects of peer-group intervention on metabolic control of adolescents with IDDM: randomized outpatient study. *Diabetes Care* 12:179–83, 1989

Cox DJ, Kovatchev BP, Julian DM, Gonder-Frederick LA, Polonsky WH, Schlundt DG, Clarke WL: Frequency of severe hypoglycemia can be predicted from self-monitoring blood glucose data. *Journal of Clinical Endocrinology and Metabolism* 79:1659–62, 1994

Delamater AM, Kurtz SC, Bubb J, White NH, Santiago JV: Self-monitoring of blood glucose by adolescents with diabetes: technical skills and utilization of data. *The Diabetes Educator* 15:56–61, 1988

Delamater AM, Bubb J, Davis S, Smith JA, White NH, Santiago JV: Randomized prospective study of self-management training with newly diagnosed diabetic children. *Diabetes Care* 13:492–98, 1990

Key #8: Social Skills

Greco P, Shroff-Pendley J, McDonell K: A peer group intervention for adolescents with type 1 diabetes and their friends. *Journal of Pediatric Psychology* 26:485–90, 2001

Gross AM, Heimann L, Shapiro R, Schultz RM: Children with diabetes: social skill training and hemoglobin A_{1C} levels. *Behavior Modification* 7:151–63, 1983

Kaplan RM, Chadwick MW, Schimmel LE: Social learning intervention to improve metabolic control in type 1 diabetes mellitus. *Diabetes Care* 8:152–55, 1985

La Greca AM, Auslander WF, Spetter D, Greco P, Skyler JS, Fisher EB, Santiago JV: I get by with a little help from my friends: adolescents' support for diabetes care. *Journal of Pediatric Psychology* 20:449–76, 1995

Key #9: Coping with School

Holmes CS: Cognitive functioning and diabetes: broadening the paradigm for behavioral and health psychology. *Diabetes Care* 10:135–36, 1987

Rovet J: Psychoeducational characteristics of children and adolescents with insulin-dependent diabetes mellitus. *Journal of Learning Disabilities* 26:7–21, 1993

Wysocki T, Harris MA, Mauras N, Fox L, Taylor A, Jackson SC, White NH: Absence of adverse effects of severe hypoglycemia on cognitive function in school-aged children with diabetes over 18 months. *Diabetes Care* 26:1100–05, 2003

Key #10: Relating to Health Professionals

Bryden KS, Peveler RC, Stein A, Neil A, Mayou RA, Dunger DB: Clinical and psychological course of diabetes from adolescence to young adulthood: a longitudinal cohort study. *Diabetes Care* 24:1536–40, 2001

Delamater AM, Kurtz SC, White NH, Santiago JV: Effects of social demand on reports of self-monitored blood glucose in adolescents with type 1 diabetes mellitus. *Journal of Applied Social Psychology* 18:491–502, 1988

Marteau TM, Johnston M, Baum JD, Bloch S: Goals of treatment in diabetes: a comparison of doctors and parents of children with diabetes. *Journal of Behavioral Medicine* 10:33–49, 1987

Wysocki T: Graduating to adult health care. *Diabetes Self Management* June:41–43, 1994

Books

American Diabetes Association: *Getting the Most Out of Diabetes Camp: A Guide for Parents and Children.* Alexandria, VA, American Diabetes Association, 2002

Betschart J, Thom S: *In Control: A Guide for Teens with Diabetes.* Minneapolis, MN, Chronimed, 1995

Brackenridge BP, Rubin RR: *Sweet Kids: How to Balance Diabetes Control and Good Nutrition with Family Peace,* 2nd ed. Alexandria, VA, American Diabetes Association, 2002

Chase HP: *Understanding Insulin-Dependent Diabetes (10th Edition).* Denver, CO, The Children's Diabetes Foundation at Denver, 2002

Geil PB, Ross TA: *Cooking Up Fun for Kids with Diabetes.* Alexandria, VA, American Diabetes Association, 2003

Lawlor M, Laffel L, Anderson BJ, Bertorelli A: *Caring for Young Children with Diabetes: Manual for Parents.* Waltham, MA, MediSense, Inc., 1996

Loring G: *Parenting a Child with Diabetes: A Practical, Empathic Guide to Help You and Your Child Live with Diabetes.* New York, McGraw Hill/Contemporary Books, 1999

Loy SN, Loy BN, Silverstein JH, Weigensberg M, Schwarzbein D: *Getting a Grip on Diabetes: Quick Tips for Kids and Teens.* Alexandria, VA, American Diabetes Association, 2000

Loy VN: *Real Life Parenting of Kids with Diabetes.* Alexandria, VA, American Diabetes Association, 1999

McAuliffe A: *Growing Up with Diabetes: What Kids Want Their Parents to Know.* New York, John Wiley and Sons, 1998

Rosenbloom AL, Silverstein JH: *Type 2 Diabetes in Children and Adolescents.* Alexandria, VA, American Diabetes Association, 2003

Siminerio L, Betschart J: *Raising a Child with Diabetes: A Guide for Parents.* Alexandria, VA, American Diabetes Association, 1995

Periodicals

Diabetes Forecast is a monthly magazine about diabetes and diabetes care for a general audience. American Diabetes Association, 1701 N. Beauregard Street, Alexandria, VA 22311 (1-800-232-3472).

Countdown is a quarterly publication of the Juvenile Diabetes Foundation oriented primarily toward updating its readers on progress in the search for a prevention and cure for type 1 diabetes. Juvenile Diabetes Research Foundation International, 120 Wall Street, New York, NY 10005-4001 (1-800-533-2873)

Diabetes Self-Management is a good source of information for those interested in intensified self-management of diabetes. Rapaport Publishing, Inc., 150 West 22nd Street, New York, NY 10011 (1-800-234-0923).

Diabetes Interview is a monthly newsletter that focuses on recent developments in the field of diabetes research and clinical practice. Kings Publishing, 6 School Street, Ste. 160, Fairfax, CA 94930-1650 (415-258-2828/1-800-488-8468)

Diabetes On-Line

There are many excellent sources of diabetes information and support available on the Internet and on the various on-line services. The larger Internet service providers often have diabetes discussion and support groups and diabetes information services that are ongoing, but details about these resources change so rapidly that it is impossible to provide specific, useful instructions to you. Most of these sources are located in the health and fitness or lifestyle sections of these services, or they can be reached by searching for a key word such as *diabetes*. There are also numerous sources of diabetes information and support available on the World Wide Web and the Internet, and these resources are increasing exponentially. One drawback is that there are no quality-control restrictions, so you must be discriminating about the faith that you put in these resources. Here is a short list of some reputable sites on the World Wide Web that you may want to try.

American Diabetes Association (ADA) is the largest organization that brings together both professionals and lay citizens to support and advocate for diabetes research, education, and treatment. You can find a quality diabetes education program that has achieved recognition in two ways: by calling your local ADA affiliate or by linking to your state's ADA affiliates home page, which is linked to ADA's home page. The ADA home page can be reached at *http://www.diabetes.org.*

National Institutes of Health, National Institute of Diabetes and Digestive and Kidney Diseases is the branch of the U.S. government that funds diabetes research. It is the most authoritative source of information on recent diabetes research. Its website also includes the Combined Health Information Database, a collection of diabetes education resources maintained by the National Diabetes Information Clearinghouse. Connect to their home page at *http://www.niddk.nih.gov/NIDDK-HomePage.html.*

Centers for Disease Control & Prevention, United States Public Health Service is the branch of the U.S. Public Health Service that is responsible for translation of recent biomedical research into clinical practice. Connect to this site at *http://www.cdc.gov/nccdphp/ddt/ddthome.html*.

Children With Diabetes is an excellent clearinghouse for all kinds of information and support specifically on childhood diabetes. Connect to their home page at *http://www.childrenwithdiabetes.com*.

American Association of Diabetes Educators (AADE) is a professional society for diabetes educators. Its home page provides information about the national certification process for diabetes educators and enables users to locate certified diabetes educators in their geographic regions. It will also provide access to on-line continuing education about diabetes for health professionals, as well as an electronic "exhibitor's area" for current information about diabetes products. The home page is linked to many of the websites listed here. Connect to the AADE home page at *http://www.AADEnet.org*.

Diabetes-Related Organizations

Here are the mailing addresses and phone numbers for major organizations concerned with diabetes. Websites are provided for those that weren't included above. Many of these organizations also have networks of state or regional chapters that can be good resources for support, information, and referrals.

American Diabetes Association
1701 N. Beauregard Street
Alexandria, VA 22311
1-800-232-3472

Juvenile Diabetes Research Foundation International
120 Wall Street
New York, NY 10005-4001
Phone: 1-800-533-CURE (2873)
Fax: 212-785-9595
http://www.jdf.org

National Diabetes Information Clearinghouse
NIH/NIDDK
1 Information Way
Bethesda, MD 20892
301-654-3327
http://diabetes.niddk.nih.gov

American Association of Diabetes Educators
100 W. Monroe
Suite 400
Chicago, IL 60603
1-800-338-3633

Mental Health Professional Organizations

American Academy of Child and Adolescent Psychiatry is the primary professional association for child and adolescent psychiatrists.

American Academy of Child and Adolescent Psychiatry
3615 Wisconsin Avenue, NW
Washington, DC 20016-3007
202-966-7300
http://www.aacap.org

American Diabetes Association, Council on Behavioral Medicine and Psychology is a subdivision of the Professional Section of ADA that fosters exchange of information among behavioral scientists regarding the psychological and behavioral aspects of diabetes. Most mental health professionals in the United States who specialize in evaluating and treating problems related to diabetes are members of this group.

Council on Behavioral Medicine and Psychology
American Diabetes Association, Professional Section
1701 N. Beauregard Street
Alexandria, VA 22311
1-800-232-3472
http://www.diabetes.org

Society of Pediatric Psychology is the primary professional organization for pediatric psychologists. It is Division 54 of the American Psychological Association.

Society of Pediatric Psychology Central Office
PO Box 170231
Atlanta, GA 30317
404-373-1099
pedpsych@aol.com
http://www.apa.org/divisions/div54/

Association for Advancement of Behavior Therapy is a professional society for mental health professionals who specialize in behavior therapy and cognitive behavior therapy techniques. Many of these professionals have experience working with patients with a variety of chronic diseases.

Association for Advancement of Behavior Therapy
305 7th Avenue, 16th Fl.,
New York, NY 10001
212-647-1890
Fax: 212-647-1865
http://www.aabt.org

Society of Developmental and Behavioral Pediatrics is a professional organization for behavioral and developmental pediatricians.

Society for Developmental and Behavioral Pediatrics
17000 Commerce Parkway, Suite C
Mt. Laurel, NJ 08054
856-439-0500
http://www.sdbp.org

INDEX

Discrimination in school, dealing
with, 141–142
Drugs, adolescents feeling pressured to
use, 130–131

E

Eating disorders, 34
Education program, evaluating your
own, 18–20
Emotional coping, 25–42
common emotional pitfalls, 28–30
critical importance of diabetes
knowledge in, 16
for fathers, 40
objectives, 28–30
promoting emotional healing,
40–42
Errors in family communication,
52–53
communicating through another
person, 53
interrupting, 53
monitoring your own, 53–54
name calling, 52
swearing, 52
yelling, 52
Evaluation
of solutions, 117–118
of your diabetes education program, 18–20
Evaluation of family communication,
50–58
communication skills, 50–52
errors, 52–53
extreme beliefs, 54–56
family structure, 56–58
self-monitoring your errors, 53–54
Exercise, in treating type 1 diabetes,
7–8

F

Fair communication, 51
Family communication, 43–62
dealing with deception, 58–60
evaluating, 50–58
teaching, 47–49
Family meetings, 60–62

Family problem-solving system,
116–119
action plan, 118
brainstorming, 117
evaluation of solutions, 117–118
problem definition, 116–117
refinement of solutions, 118
verification, 117
Family sharing of diabetes responsibilities, 63–80
acquiring skills, 66–67
Diabetes Independence Survey,
67–73
for fathers, 79–80
steps toward independence, 67
teaching about long-term complications, 77–78
transferring diabetes responsibilities
to your child, 73–76
Family structure, 56–58
adolescent involvement in marital
discord, 57–58
cross-generational coalitions, 57
triangulation, 57
weak parental coalitions, 57
Fat (dietary), 7
Fathers
diabetes knowledge for, 21–22
emotional coping for, 40
family sharing of diabetes responsibilities for, 79–80
stress management for, 89
Fights, scheduling, 50–51
Food and Drug Administration, 122

G

Glucose testing, 102–103
continuous sensors for, 15
in treating type 1 diabetes, 6
Grieving process, 30

H

Healing, emotional, 40–42
Health care
children as consumers of, 151–156
transition to adult, 157–158